COMPACT *Research*

Diabetes

by Janice M. Yuwiler

Diseases and Disorders

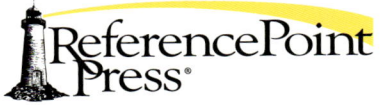

San Diego, CA

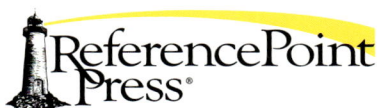

© 2010 ReferencePoint Press, Inc.

For more information, contact:
ReferencePoint Press, Inc.
PO Box 27779
San Diego, CA 92198
www.ReferencePointPress.com

ALL RIGHTS RESERVED.
No part of this work covered by the copyright hereon may be reproduced or used in any form or by any means—graphic, electronic, or mechanical, including photocopying, recording, taping, Web distribution, or information storage retrieval systems—without the written permission of the publisher.

Picture credits:
Cover: iStockphoto.com
Maury Aaseng: 31–33, 45–47, 60–63, 75–77
AP Images: 15
iStockphoto.com: 11

LIBRARY OF CONGRESS CATALOGING-IN-PUBLICATION DATA

Yuwiler, Janice M.
　Diabetes / by Janice M. Yuwiler.
　　p. cm. — (Compact research)
　Includes bibliographical references and index.
　ISBN-13: 978-1-60152-076-0 (hardback)
　ISBN-10: 1-60152-076-X (hardback)
　1. Diabetes—Popular works. I. Title.
RC660.4.Y89 2009
616.4'62—dc22

2009006173

Contents

Foreword	4
Diabetes at a Glance	6
Overview	8
How Serious Is Diabetes?	20
Primary Source Quotes	27
Facts and Illustrations	30
What Causes Diabetes?	34
Primary Source Quotes	41
Facts and Illustrations	44
How Is Diabetes Treated?	48
Primary Source Quotes	55
Facts and Illustrations	59
Can Diabetes Be Cured?	64
Primary Source Quotes	71
Facts and Illustrations	74
Key People and Advocacy Groups	78
Chronology	82
Related Organizations	84
For Further Research	88
Source Notes	90
List of Illustrations	92
Index	93
About the Author	96

Foreword

> "Where is the knowledge we have lost in information?"
>
> —T.S. Eliot, "The Rock."

As modern civilization continues to evolve, its ability to create, store, distribute, and access information expands exponentially. The explosion of information from all media continues to increase at a phenomenal rate. By 2020 some experts predict the worldwide information base will double every 73 days. While access to diverse sources of information and perspectives is paramount to any democratic society, information alone cannot help people gain knowledge and understanding. Information must be organized and presented clearly and succinctly in order to be understood. The challenge in the digital age becomes not the creation of information, but how best to sort, organize, enhance, and present information.

ReferencePoint Press developed the *Compact Research* series with this challenge of the information age in mind. More than any other subject area today, researching current issues can yield vast, diverse, and unqualified information that can be intimidating and overwhelming for even the most advanced and motivated researcher. The *Compact Research* series offers a compact, relevant, intelligent, and conveniently organized collection of information covering a variety of current topics ranging from illegal immigration and deforestation to diseases such as anorexia and meningitis.

The series focuses on three types of information: objective single-author narratives, opinion-based primary source quotations, and facts and statistics. The clearly written objective narratives provide context and reliable background information. Primary source quotes are carefully selected and cited, exposing the reader to differing points of view. And facts and statistics sections aid the reader in evaluating perspectives. Presenting these key types of information creates a richer, more balanced learning experience.

For better understanding and convenience, the series enhances information by organizing it into narrower topics and adding design features that make it easy for a reader to identify desired content. For example, in *Compact Research: Illegal Immigration*, a chapter covering the economic impact of illegal immigration has an objective narrative explaining the various ways the economy is impacted, a balanced section of numerous primary source quotes on the topic, followed by facts and full-color illustrations to encourage evaluation of contrasting perspectives.

The ancient Roman philosopher Lucius Annaeus Seneca wrote, "It is quality rather than quantity that matters." More than just a collection of content, the *Compact Research* series is simply committed to creating, finding, organizing, and presenting the most relevant and appropriate amount of information on a current topic in a user-friendly style that invites, intrigues, and fosters understanding.

Diabetes at a Glance

Prevalence
America is currently experiencing an epidemic of diabetes. In 2007 more than 23.6 million people in the United States had diabetes, which is a leading cause of death in the nation.

Prognosis
Diabetes is a deadly disease that can be controlled with medication, diet, and exercise. Poorly controlled diabetes can lead to death and disability, including blindness, kidney failure, stroke, heart attack, nerve damage, and amputation.

Type 1 Diabetes
Type 1 diabetes mostly strikes children and adolescents and is a lifelong disease. People with type 1 diabetes must take daily injections of insulin or they will die.

Type 2 Diabetes
Type 2 diabetes mostly occurs among people who are over age 40, overweight, and inactive, but it is becoming more common in young adults and teens. New research indicates type 2 diabetes may be preventable.

Metabolic Syndrome
Also called syndrome X, metabolic syndrome is a cluster of risk factors for diabetes and heart disease. Associated with higher-than-normal blood

sugar levels, belly fat, and high blood pressure, metabolic syndrome is becoming more common as the rate of childhood obesity skyrockets.

Treatment

Medication and lifestyle changes are the primary means of treating diabetes. People with type 1 diabetes must take daily insulin injections. Most people with type 2 diabetes take oral medications. Weight loss and exercise can help control type 2 diabetes.

Finding a Cure

At present there is no cure for diabetes, although researchers continue to explore organ transplants, the use of stem cells, and the creation of an artificial pancreas.

Prevention

Weight loss and exercise can prevent and even reverse type 2 diabetes. There is currently no known way to prevent type 1 diabetes, but the severe consequences of the disease can be prevented through careful monitoring of blood sugar levels combined with a daily juggle of insulin, food, and exercise.

Overview

❝Every day, all day, I take care of people with diabetes. My patients come in all shapes and sizes, ethnicities and ages. I see the success stories and the chronic problems. . . . On the same day I see a fifty-six-year-old diabetes-related double amputee in a wheelchair I may see a seventy-six-year-old, who has had diabetes since the 1940s, who never misses his daily four-mile walk with his dog.❞

—Anne L. Peters, director of the University of Southern California's clinical diabetes programs.

❝Diabetes sucks! It's that it's everyday. No matter what. Wherever I go, I've got diabetes.❞

—Gordon, age 15, diagnosed with type 1 diabetes.

What Is Diabetes?

Diabetes is an ancient and deadly disease—a metabolic disorder. People with diabetes have trouble processing the food they eat, especially carbohydrates. The problem begins when food is broken down in the intestines into its core components and large amounts of glucose, a simple sugar, enter the bloodstream. Normally, the body has a system of checks and balances that monitor the amount of glucose available in the blood for the cells to use. If there is too little glucose in the blood, glycogen from the liver is converted to glucose for the cells' use. If there is too much sugar in the blood, the pancreas boosts production of a hormone called insulin to move sugar into the cells. In this way the body maintains an adequate level of glucose in the blood.

For people with diabetes the system of checks and balances does not work. Glucose does not enter the cells properly, and sugar builds up in the blood. The kidneys struggle to remove the excess sugar from the blood but are soon overwhelmed. Sugar spills into the urine, creating the classic signs of diabetes: sugar in the urine and frequent urination. It is the sugar in the urine that gives diabetes its scientific name, diabetes mellitus, which means the "honey diabetes."

Lack of Insulin

Insulin is a hormone produced by the pancreas. The pancreas is a soft, spongy organ that is part of the human digestive system. It is shaped somewhat like a banana and located behind the stomach at the level of the navel. The pancreas produces a number of substances that are crucial to the body's ability to digest food. The bulk of the pancreas is made up of acinar cells that produce digestive juices funneled through ducts to the small intestine. But scattered throughout the acinar cells are little islands of cells of another kind. These are called the islets of Langerhans, after their discoverer, German medical student Paul Langerhans.

The islets of Langerhans are made up of three different types of cells: alpha, beta, and delta cells. All three types of cells produce hormones that control the body's use of sugar. The beta cells produce the hormone insulin. Insulin binds to cell membranes and allows glucose to enter the cells. It is similar to a lock and key mechanism. Insulin functions as the key to open the door to the cells. Without insulin, glucose cannot enter a cell and be used for energy.

> **For people with diabetes the system of checks and balances does not work. Glucose does not enter the cells properly, and sugar builds up in the blood.**

The amount of glucose present in the blood triggers the beta cells to produce more or less insulin as needed to maintain the body's blood sugar within a certain range. For people with diabetes, this mechanism does not work. Either insulin is not produced in sufficient quantities or it does not work properly, and blood sugar levels climb.

Types of Diabetes

There are two main types of diabetes. Type 1 diabetes is the most severe form. People with type 1 diabetes do not produce insulin and must have daily injections of insulin to survive. According to physician Stanley Mirsky: "Type 1 diabetes generally shows up very abruptly and dramatically, with unmistakable symptoms—excessive urination and thirst, dramatic weight loss, weakness, irritability. If these symptoms go untreated, they rapidly progress into acidosis [severely unbalanced pH] and finally coma in only a few days or weeks."[1] Type 1 diabetes most frequently occurs among children and young adults, with about 1 in every 400 to 500 children having type 1 diabetes.

> **More than 90 percent of the people with diabetes in the United States have type 2 diabetes. People with type 2 diabetes continue to produce insulin, but their bodies are resistant to insulin's effects.**

Type 2 diabetes is the most common type of diabetes. More than 90 percent of the people with diabetes in the United States have type 2 diabetes. People with type 2 diabetes continue to produce insulin, but their bodies are resistant to insulin's effects. Because the body is still producing insulin, type 2 diabetes can often be controlled without injections of insulin. Instead, oral medications can be used either to increase the amount of insulin produced by the pancreas or to help insulin bind to the cell membranes and allow glucose to enter the cells. In addition, some people with type 2 diabetes can control the disease by losing excess weight, exercising, eating a healthy diet, and monitoring their blood sugar.

Unlike type 1 diabetes, type 2 diabetes often occurs gradually without obvious warning signs. Symptoms can include frequent urination, excessive thirst, blurred vision, fatigue, depression, and sores that do not heal. Type 2 diabetes occurs mainly in adults over the age of 40 who are overweight and inactive.

Overview

How Serious Is Diabetes?

The problem of diabetes is growing. The Centers for Disease Control and Prevention estimate that 1 in 3 children born in the year 2000 will develop diabetes in their lifetimes. Currently, almost 8 percent of the U.S. population has diabetes. Of that 8 percent, 17.9 million people know they have the disease, but 5.7 million people, almost a fourth of those with the disease, are undiagnosed. Without treatment, these people will die. Even with treatment, people with diabetes are at twice the risk of death. Diabetes is routinely among the leading causes of death in the United States.

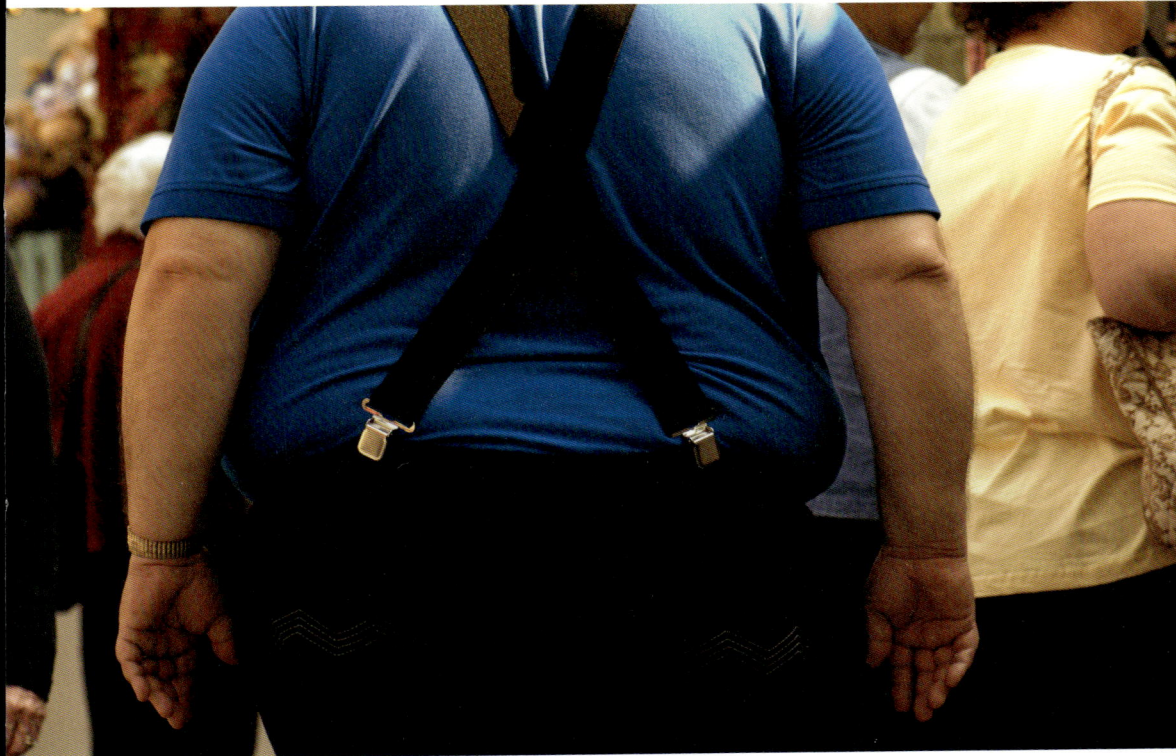

In 2007 more than 23.6 million people in the United States had diabetes, which is a leading cause of death in the United States. Maintaining normal weight and getting moderate exercise has been proven to prevent or delay the onset of diabetes in people at high risk for the disease. Losing 5 to 7 percent of body weight and exercising 30 minutes most days were enough to make a difference.

Diabetes

The chance of getting diabetes varies by type. Those most at risk for type 2 diabetes include people who are over age 45, overweight, inactive, and have a parent, brother, or sister with diabetes. African Americans, Native Americans, Hispanics, and Pacific Islanders are at particular risk for getting type 2 diabetes.

Type 1 diabetes is less common and typically strikes children and adolescents. These young people are usually thin to normal weight. If there is a strong history of type 1 diabetes in the family, other children in the family are at greater risk for getting the disease.

Complications

Francine Ratner Kaufman, past president of the American Diabetes Association, notes: "Diabetes is relentless and the complications are terrible. . . . I'm talking about blindness, heart attacks, strokes, kidney failure, and amputations."[2] In the short term, uncontrolled diabetes can cause loss of consciousness and death. Over time, diabetes can lead to blindness, nerve damage, heart disease, kidney failure, and amputation.

Among those with type 1 diabetes, 35 percent will die of a fatal heart attack by age 55. Kidney failure is common, and nearly everyone with type 1 diabetes will suffer eye damage after 20 years with the disease. More than 60 percent of those with type 2 diabetes will also have eye damage after living with diabetes for 20 years. The damage leads, most often, to mild vision problems, although diabetes is also the leading cause of blindness for people between the ages of 20 and 74 years.

> **In the short term, uncontrolled diabetes can cause loss of consciousness and death. Over time, diabetes can lead to blindness, nerve damage, heart disease, kidney failure, and amputation.**

High blood sugar levels caused by diabetes lead to a loss of circulation and an increased risk of infections. People with diabetes tend to heal slowly, and 60 to 65 percent have high blood pressure. Diabetes also increases the risk for stroke, heart attacks, and kidney failure. In over 40 percent of patients with kidney failure, the cause is diabetes.

What Causes Diabetes?

The causes of type 1 and type 2 diabetes are different. Type 1 diabetes is an autoimmune disease. For some reason the person's immune system seeks out and destroys the beta cells in the pancreas, leaving the person unable to produce insulin. The autoimmune reaction occurs mainly in non-Hispanic white children aged 8 to 18 years, and the cause is unknown. Scientists believe the autoimmune reaction might be due to a genetic susceptibility that is triggered by a virus or toxin in the environment.

Type 2 diabetes tends to run in families, with American Indians, African Americans, Hispanic/Latino Americans, and Asians/Pacific Islanders most at risk for the disease. The theory is that members of these populations have a "thrifty gene," or the ability to survive on little food. If excess food is consumed and people gain weight, they increase their risk of developing type 2 diabetes, especially if they store fat around their middle. Although the body continues to produce insulin as a person gains weight, there is the risk that the pancreas will wear out over time as it tries to keep up with the increased demand for insulin. In addition, large amounts of belly fat appear to produce chemicals that decrease the body's ability to use insulin. Most people who develop type 2 diabetes are over age 40, overweight, and are not physically active.

> **Those patients who kept their blood sugar levels strictly within the normal range suffered far fewer of the health complications associated with diabetes.**

Childhood Obesity

Obesity, one of the leading risk factors for type 2 diabetes, has increased nationwide by 50 percent in the last decade. Nearly 15 percent of children and teens in the United States are overweight and will likely grow up to be overweight adults. Experts fear that the epidemic of childhood obesity in the United States could lead to large numbers of young adults developing type 2 diabetes. In fact, recent studies show a dramatic increase in type 2 diabetes among people in their twenties and thirties. As feared, what used to be a disease of midlife to old age is now affecting younger people.

Diabetes

Joyce Lee, a pediatric endocrinologist at the University of Michigan's Mott Children's Hospital, warns: "The full impact of the childhood obesity epidemic has yet to be seen because it can take up to ten years or longer for obese individuals to develop type 2 diabetes. Children who are obese today are more likely to develop type 2 diabetes as young adults."[3] The risks are so great that the American Academy of Pediatrics has developed new screening guidelines and treatment recommendations to identify and treat overweight children in order to reduce their risk for type 2 diabetes. And Lee, among others, is calling for obesity prevention and treatment in schools, communities, and the health-care system.

How Is Diabetes Treated?

"Daily monitoring and careful control of blood sugar levels are the most important steps that people with diabetes can take,"[4] says David G. Orloff, former director of the Food and Drug Administration's Division of Metabolic and Endocrine Drugs. The importance of maintaining near-normal blood sugar levels was demonstrated by the 10-year Diabetes Control and Complications Trial that tracked almost 1,500 men, women, and teens with type 1 diabetes from 1983 to 1993. Those patients who kept their blood sugar levels strictly within the normal range suffered far fewer of the health complications associated with diabetes. Their risk of eye damage decreased by 76 percent, nerve damage fell by 60 percent, and the progression of their diabetes slowed by 54 percent.

> **Continuous glucose monitoring systems are inserted under the skin and record how a person's blood sugar varies throughout the day, allowing the user to adjust insulin, food, or exercise in response to changes in the blood sugar level.**

Controlling blood sugar requires frequent testing of blood sugar levels and responding as needed with insulin, food, exercise, or changes in medication. To test blood sugar, a person pricks the side of a finger with a lancet (which is a small, sharp medical blade) to produce a single drop of blood. The drop of blood

Overview

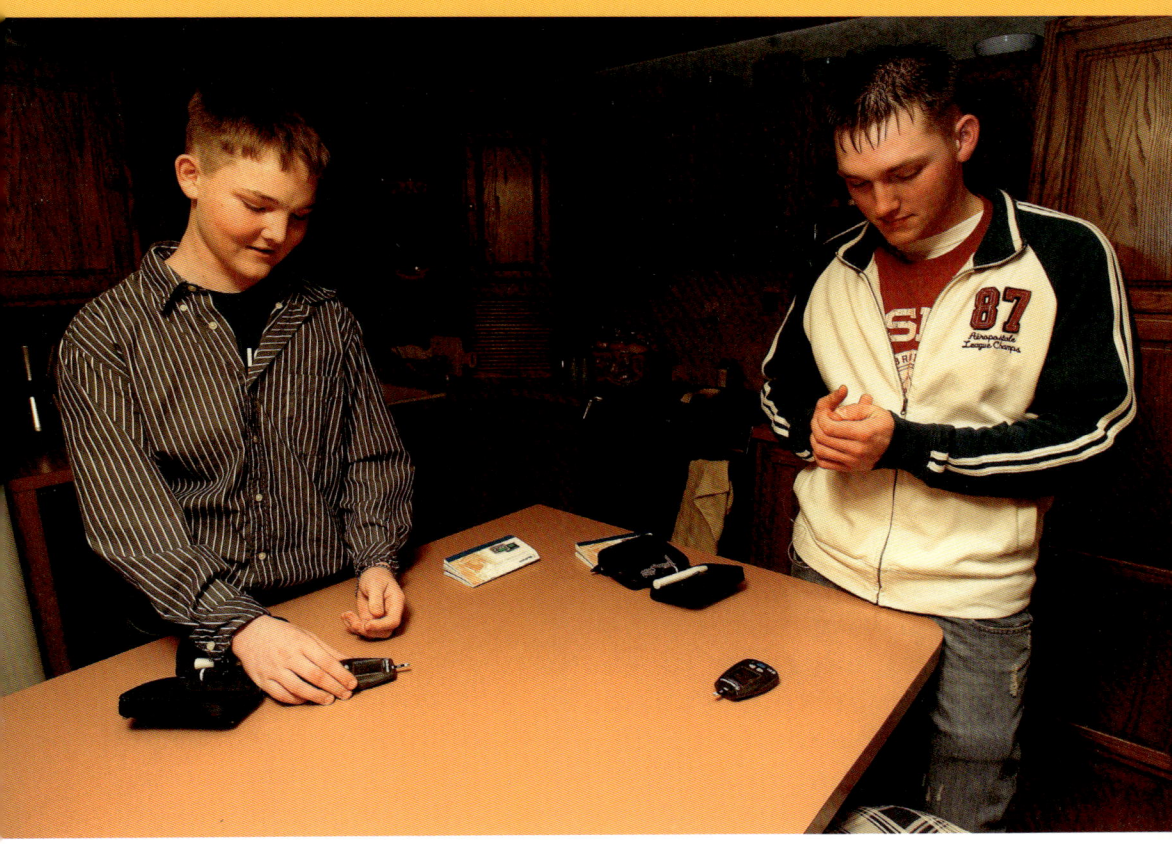

Type 1 diabetes mostly strikes children and adolescents and is a lifelong disease. People with type 1 diabetes must take daily injections of insulin or they will die. These young men, both of whom have type 1 diabetes, monitor their blood sugar.

is smeared onto a strip of specially formulated paper, and the paper inserted into a machine called a blood glucose monitor. Most blood glucose monitors are easily portable, the size of a cell phone, and quickly calculate and display a person's blood sugar level. However, nothing can replace the minute-by-minute monitoring of blood sugar performed by the body. Oral medications, insulin injections, food choices, and exercise all help to regulate the body's blood sugar level, but they do not offer perfect control.

A healthy pancreas releases a low level of insulin continuously. When blood sugar rises after a meal, the pancreas produces more insulin. When insulin levels are low, the liver releases glycogen to nourish the cells and to keep blood sugar within a tightly controlled range. People with diabetes must mimic this system via oral medications and insulin.

Those with type 1 diabetes need insulin to replace the insulin their bodies cannot produce. Insulin does not come in pill form. It must be injected, typically several times a day. It is the timing of the injections and the amount of insulin injected that are crucial. Too much insulin can lead to a drop in blood sugar and diabetic coma. Too little insulin results in high blood sugar and complications of the disease. The use of long-acting and short-acting insulins helps achieve the proper balance, but the balance must be constantly monitored by checking blood sugar levels.

While some people with type 2 diabetes use insulin, most use oral medications, food choices, and exercise to control their blood sugar. Of the three main types of medication used, all strive to make use of the insulin the pancreas still produces. One type stimulates beta cells in the pancreas to produce more insulin. A second keeps blood sugar levels down by reducing the amount of glucose released by the liver between meals and helping the cells bind to the insulin that is available. And a third works to slow the digestion of carbohydrates so that glucose is released slowly into the bloodstream, rather than all at once after a meal.

> **Maintaining normal weight and getting moderate exercise has been proven to prevent or delay the onset of diabetes in people at high risk for the disease.**

New Technologies

Recent developments in technology have improved the lives of thousands of people with diabetes. Slimmer lancets and laser lancets reduce the pain of the required finger stick. All-in-one blood sugar monitors take blood from an arm or thigh, which is less painful, and transfer and analyze the blood in one seamless process. There is a wristwatch monitor that detects blood sugar levels under the skin and sounds an alarm if the blood sugar level is too high or too low. Continuous glucose monitoring systems are inserted under the skin and record how a person's blood sugar varies throughout the day, allowing the user to adjust insulin, food, or exercise in response to changes in the blood sugar level.

Improvements have also been made in the delivery of insulin. Insulin now comes in short- and long-lasting forms. Thinner needles make injections less painful, insulin jet injectors use air pressure to send a fine spray of insulin through the skin, a form of inhaled insulin has recently come on the market, and insulin pen injectors (they look like a cartridge pen) offer a way to transport and inject insulin that is simple and discreet.

> "Advances in medication and technology continue to make diabetes management easier and more effective."

In addition, insulin pumps are becoming more common. Worn outside the body like a pager, the pump continuously provides insulin through a catheter inserted under the skin of the abdomen. The constant infusion of insulin mimics the work of the pancreas. The user increases the dose of insulin before meals and adjusts the level of insulin when exercising. When combined with close monitoring of blood sugar, an insulin pump can maintain normal to near-normal blood sugar levels. Insulin pumps are now being paired with continuous glucose monitors to provide control that comes ever closer to mimicking the natural response of the pancreas to blood sugar levels.

Can Diabetes Be Cured?

Advancements in surgical techniques and the rise of genetic engineering bring new hope for a cure. Since 1966 surgeons have performed pancreas transplants, usually in conjunction with a kidney transplant. If it works, the new pancreas produces insulin and cures the patient's diabetes. But there are few pancreases available for transplant, and the potential for organ rejection requires the use of antirejection drugs for life. These drugs often have side effects that are worse than taking insulin.

In addition, investigation continues into harvesting and transplanting the islets of Langerhans instead of the entire pancreas. It is a simpler surgery, and in one study 70 to 80 percent of the patients had normal blood sugar levels following the procedure without the use of insulin.

But the islets with their beta cells seem to erode over time. Only 11 percent of the patients still had normal blood sugar levels five years later. Furthermore, islet transplantation is haunted by the same problems as pancreas transplants: a lack of pancreases from which to obtain the islets and the need for antirejection drugs.

Other hopes for a cure rest with the creation of an artificial or biomechanical pancreas. By combining insulin pump technology, a continuous glucose monitor, and a device that interfaces between the two, it may be possible to develop a mechanical device that performs the function of a healthy pancreas. The necessary computer programs are currently being tested. In addition, efforts continue to focus on producing new beta cells that could be inserted into the body and survive the autoimmune process that killed the original beta cells. And startling new research in mice hints at a way to stop a patient's autoimmune response to transplanted beta cells and allow the pancreas to regenerate functioning beta cells on its own.

Prevention

Perhaps the best hope for a cure for future generations is prevention. New cases of type 2 diabetes occur most frequently among people who are overweight and inactive. Maintaining normal weight and getting moderate exercise has been proven to prevent or delay the onset of diabetes in people at high risk for the disease. Losing 5 to 7 percent of body weight and exercising 30 minutes most days were enough to make a difference. As Jaime Torres of the National Hispanic Medical Association says, "Everything counts—taking the stairs, walking the dog, dancing to music, mowing the lawn . . . physical activity just needs to occur every day."[5]

Preventing type 1 diabetes is less straightforward. Recent clinical trials funded by the National Institutes of Health failed to prevent type 1 diabetes in high-risk patients. Neither insulin nor oral diabetic medication prevented the onset of type 1 diabetes. The most promising hope to limit type 1 diabetes is an antibody called anti-CD3. When given to patients recently diagnosed with type 1 diabetes, anti-CD3 seems to prevent further destruction of the beta cells, leaving patients able to produce some insulin on their own. According to Kevan Herold of Columbia University, who conducted one of the clinical trials, "The clinical effect we saw persisted long after patients had finished treatment with the anti-

CD3 antibody."[6] Larger clinical trials are under way with the hope that rapid treatment might prevent complete destruction of the beta cells and a lifelong dependence on insulin.

In the meantime, advances in medication and technology continue to make diabetes management easier and more effective. Efforts are being made to educate the public and promote lifestyle changes that will reduce the incidence of type 2 diabetes. And those living with diabetes and their families follow the latest in scientific research hoping a cure will be found.

How Serious Is Diabetes?

> **I try to explain, but how do you convey the enormity of a chronic, life-threatening disease to a three-year-old? How do you say that he will have to take insulin for the rest of his life, that he will be denied many foods, that he may pass out from low blood sugar, and that every organ in his body is now at risk?**
>
> —James S. Hirsch, diagnosed with diabetes at age 15, upon learning his son has type 1 diabetes.

> **The most important thing you can do to deal with diabetes is to make every miniscule attempt to take every possible opportunity to MAKE LIFE A LITTLE BETTER. Don't live with what you've been dealt. Fight back. Make it better.**
>
> —Chuck Eichten, who has successfully controlled his type 1 diabetes for over 25 years.

Sitting in a wheelchair, her face drooping on one side from a prior stroke, the elderly woman living in downtown Los Angeles answered the doctor's questions about her diabetes. "They told me I had the sugar in 1966. They took my foot in 1987. Gangrene." In 1990 she had a mild heart attack, and then a stroke in 1993. The stroke affected her left leg and arm. Her arm was still paralyzed. "I been going to therapy for two years pretty regular. Still I can't open my hand. . . . Everybody has a little bit of the sugar in our family, 'cept my daughter here."[7]

Three generations were sitting in the doctor's office that day. At age 13, her granddaughter had just been diagnosed with type 2 diabetes. But

How Serious Is Diabetes?

this time, the story might be different. Unlike the grandmother, the teenager's mother was determined to fight the disease. "My whole life, I've watched diabetes eat my mother to pieces because she doesn't take care of herself. No way will I let that happen to [my daughter]."[8]

Diabetes kills. Quickly if the body produces no insulin (type 1 diabetes), or more slowly for those with type 2 diabetes, whose bodies still produce some insulin. Either way, excess sugar in the blood attacks all organs of the body, causing blindness, sores that do not heal, nerve damage, kidney damage, and increased risk of heart attacks and strokes. With the use of insulin, new medications, lifestyle changes, and advances in technology, diabetes can be controlled and managed, but it takes work.

How Common Is Diabetes?

The number of people with diabetes in the United States is growing at an alarming rate. Tommy Thompson, U.S. secretary of health and human services from 2001 to 2005, warned, "[The country] risks being overwhelmed by the health and human consequences of an ever-growing diabetes epidemic."[9] In fact, the National Diabetes Information Clearinghouse estimates that in 2007, 23.6 million people had diabetes in the United States, or 7.8 percent of the U.S. population. Of those, about 25 percent, or 5.7 million people, are undiagnosed—they do not know they have diabetes, and because they are not receiving treatment they are at risk of suffering the disease's devastating effects.

Type 1 diabetes usually strikes children and young adults, although it can occur at any age. Non-Hispanic white children are most at risk. In the United States in 2007 about 186,300 youth younger than age 20 had diabetes. Most of them had type 1 diabetes. In contrast, only 5 to 10 percent of adults diagnosed with diabetes each year are diagnosed with type 1 diabetes.

Type 2 diabetes accounts for 90 to 95 percent of all cases of newly

> **Excess sugar in the blood attacks all organs of the body, causing blindness, sores that do not heal, nerve damage, kidney damage, and increased risk of heart attacks and strokes.**

diagnosed diabetes among adults in the United States. In 2007 alone 1.6 million new cases of diabetes were diagnosed among people aged 20 or older. Most of the new cases had type 2 diabetes, with African Americans, Hispanic/Latino Americans, American Indians, and Asians/Pacific Islanders most at risk for the disease.

In addition, at least 57 million additional Americans over age 19 in 2007 had prediabetes. In other words, they had blood sugar levels higher than normal, but not high enough to be diagnosed as having diabetes. These 57 million Americans are at risk for developing diabetes, heart disease, and stroke.

What Does Diabetes Cost?

Diabetes is expensive. Daily management of diabetes includes the cost of insulin and syringes, oral medication, test strips to test blood sugar, and devices such as blood glucose monitors and insulin pumps. There are also the costs of treating complications of diabetes. In 2007 the American Diabetes Association estimated the total cost of diabetes as $174 billion. Of that amount, $116 billion is for medical expenses. About 61 percent of the medical costs are spent on hospital care and medications to treat complications of diabetes, including heart and kidney disease, nerve damage, and problems due to poor circulation.

Living with Diabetes

Managing diabetes takes effort but it can be done. Typically it requires sticking to a schedule, with meals timed to coincide with the peak effect of insulin injections and enduring the inconvenience and pain of pricking a finger to test the level of sugar in the blood. If the blood sugar level is low, eating a snack will correct the problem. If the blood sugar level is high, exercise or an injection of insulin will bring the blood sugar level down. People who are in control of their diabetes typically test their blood sugar not just once, but several times a day and adjust their food intake, exercise, and amount of insulin accordingly. People with type 2 diabetes have the best results when they lose weight and exercise at least 30 minutes a day.

Keeping blood sugar levels close to normal can prevent the long-term complications of diabetes, but it requires daily monitoring. NFL quarterback Jay Cutler, who has type 1 diabetes, says, "Diabetes is the toughest opponent I've ever faced, but I wasn't going to let it slow down my career. And kids don't have to let it stop them from reaching for their dreams."[10]

William H. Polonsky, a psychologist at the University of California, San Diego, comments on the frustrations that can build in people who must cope daily with diabetes. "Living with diabetes can be terribly frustrating and difficult. It is not just a simple matter of eating right or taking your medications properly. Diabetes is often an emotional struggle as well. Some [diabetics] are infuriated with diabetes, some depressed. Others are frightened, frustrated, guilt-ridden, or in denial."[11] Yet with support and access to appropriate medication and technology, diabetes can be managed, allowing people with the disease to live long and active lives.

Complications of Diabetes

As N.R. Kleinfield reported in the *New York Times:* "Diabetes has no cure. It is progressive and often fatal, and while the patient lives, the welter of medical complications it sets off can attack every major organ."[12] The problem is that extra sugar in the blood gets carried throughout the body. Over time the excess sugar causes damage to the eyes, nerves, blood vessels, and kidneys, among other organs. The immune system is affected, so bacterial and fungal infections become more common. Almost one-third of people with diabetes have gum disease, and cuts and sores heal slowly, leading to amputation of toes, feet, or legs if gangrene sets in. As many as 71,000 lower-limb amputations are done in the United States each year as a result of complications of diabetes.

> **While diabetes can be managed, there is the inconvenience and pain of pricking a finger to test the level of sugar in the blood.**

About 60 to 70 percent of people with diabetes suffer some degree of nerve damage, including numbness, slowed digestion, problems with bladder control, sexual dysfunction, and prickling, tingling, burning, aching, or pain in the arms and legs. Florene Linnen, a community advocate for better control of diabetes, recalls a woman whose feet were so numb from the impact of her diabetes that when walking on hot pavement she did not realize the bottom of her feet were getting burned. She later had to have both feet amputated.

Changes to the Blood Vessels

Diabetes causes a gradual thickening and narrowing of blood vessels, slowing blood flow and causing high blood pressure, heart disease, stroke, and poor circulation. A study found that 75 percent of adults with diabetes had high blood pressure or were taking medication for high blood pressure. And the risk of heart disease and stroke is two to four times greater in people with diabetes than those without the disease.

High blood pressure in combination with high blood sugar often damages the kidneys, making diabetes the leading cause of kidney failure. If the kidneys fail, long-term dialysis or a kidney transplant is needed for the person to survive. In 2005 a total of 178,689 people with end-stage kidney disease due to diabetes were living via dialysis or a kidney transplant. John Chalmers, one of the coprincipal investigators of a large study looking at high blood pressure and high blood sugar, says:

> Protecting the kidney[s] is extremely important for patients with diabetes because it's one of the main complications. It's terrifying, and leads in the long term to dialysis, renal [kidney] transplantation and death. Secondly, it's a marker for all the other things in diabetes. Having protein in the urine and developing kidney disease is an indication that a person with diabetes may end up having a stroke or a heart attack.[13]

Changes in the blood vessels caused by diabetes also affect the blood vessels at the back of the eye. If blood vessels in the retina bulge and leak blood, they can damage the eye, causing blurry vision or blindness. Most people who have had diabetes for 20 years will have some damage to their eyes, although it may not progress to blindness.

An Epidemic of Type 2 Diabetes

The number of people suffering from diabetes has skyrocketed over the past 50 years. In 1985 an estimated 30 million people had diabetes worldwide. By 2000 the number of people worldwide with diabetes had grown to 177 million, and the number is estimated to rise to 370 mil-

How Serious Is Diabetes?

lion by 2030. Almost all of the increase is due to new cases of type 2 diabetes in an ever-increasing overweight and inactive population throughout the world.

Over 80 percent of people with type 2 diabetes are overweight or obese. The office of the surgeon general reports that a weight gain of 11 to 18 pounds (5 to 8.2kg) doubles a person's risk of getting type 2 diabetes. "Both adults and children are eating too much, exercising too little, and getting fatter,"[14] says physician Boyd E. Metzger, writing for the American Medical Association. Today many people drive everywhere, eat fast foods laden with fat and served in ever-larger portions, and work at desk or other sedentary jobs. The result is an epidemic of diabetes in the United States and the world.

The impact is reflected in the experience of the people of the island of Nauru in the central Pacific. Until the 1950s Nauruans lived off subsistence farming and fishing. Obesity and diabetes were virtually unknown. In the 1960s, the Nauruans realized the value of the island's soil, which foreign companies had been selling for fertilizer. The Nauruans took control of the business and began profiting from it. By 1976 the people of Nauru were among the wealthiest in the world. Farming and fishing disappeared in a generation. Cars, imported foods, electric appliances, and televisions became commonplace. The change in lifestyle was dramatic. By 1976 the average Nauruan was obese, and 34.4 percent of the population had diabetes.

> **About 60 to 70 percent of people with diabetes suffer some degree of nerve damage, including numbness, slowed digestion, problems with bladder control, sexual dysfunction, and prickling, tingling, burning, aching, or pain in the arms and legs.**

The experience of the Nauruans is echoed in New York City. Kleinfield of the *New York Times* reports: "An estimated 800,000 adult New Yorkers—more than one in every eight—now have diabetes, and city health officials describe the problem as a bona fide epidemic. Diabetes is the only major disease in the city that is growing . . . and it's growing quickly even as other scourges like heart disease and cancers are stable or on the decline."[15] The experience is not limited to New York City. The incidence of diabetes is growing throughout the United States.

Young People at Risk

The number of young adults hospitalized with diabetes in the United States has increased along with the rate of childhood obesity. According to Joyce Lee at the University of Michigan's Mott's Children's Hospital: "Today's young adults experienced childhood and adolescence in the leading edge of the childhood obesity epidemic in the 1970s and 1980s. Our findings suggest that we may now just be beginning to see the first manifestation of a related 'diabetes epidemic' among these young adults."[16] In the United States type 2 diabetes is rapidly shifting from being a disease of those 40 and above to being a disease of young people as well.

> **Today many people drive everywhere, eat fast foods laden with fat and served in ever-larger portions, and work at desk or other sedentary jobs. The result is an epidemic of diabetes in the United States and the world.**

The longer a person lives with diabetes, the more likely he or she is to suffer the consequences of diabetes, including blindness, amputations, nerve damage, kidney failure, and heart disease. This means that a young adult with type 2 diabetes is more likely to develop complications during his or her lifetime than people who develop diabetes when they are older. The full effect will not be known for years, but doctors fear that within a generation or two, huge waves of people suffering the consequences of diabetes could overwhelm the health-care system.

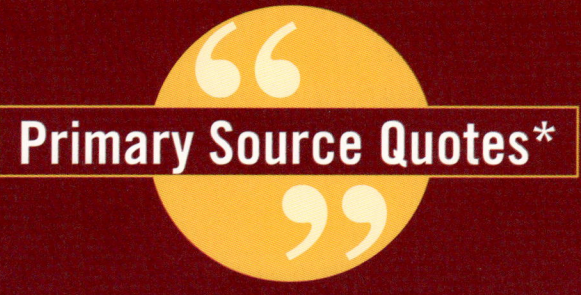

Primary Source Quotes*

How Serious Is Diabetes?

66 **The pandemic of obesity, diabetes, and heart disease, based on changes in lifestyle, poses the greatest threat to our survival for the foreseeable future.** 99

—David M. Nathan and Linda M. Delahanty, *Beating Diabetes: The First Complete Program Clinically Proven to Dramatically Improve Your Glucose Tolerance*. New York: McGraw-Hill, 2005.

Nathan is a professor of medicine at Harvard Medical School and director of the Diabetes Center at Massachusetts General Hospital. Delahanty is chief dietitian and director of nutrition and behavioral research at the Diabetes Center at Massachusetts General Hospital.

66 **Diabetes is America's most common and costly chronic illness, touching all segments of society while ravaging minority communities in particular.** 99

—James S. Hirsch. *Cheating Destiny: Living with Diabetes*. Boston: Houghton Mifflin, 2006.

Hirsch is a former reporter for the *New York Times* and the *Wall Street Journal*. Hirsch was diagnosed with type 1 diabetes at age 15 and has a son and brother who also have type 1 diabetes.

---

* Editor's Note: While the definition of a primary source can be narrowly or broadly defined, for the purposes of Compact Research, a primary source consists of: 1) results of original research presented by an organization or researcher; 2) eyewitness accounts of events, personal experience, or work experience; 3) first-person editorials offering pundits' opinions; 4) government officials presenting political plans and/or policies; 5) representatives of organizations presenting testimony or policy.

Diabetes

> "The diabetes epidemic in the United States continues unabated, with a staggering toll in acute and chronic complications, disability, and death."

—Robert Steinbrook, "Facing the Diabetes Epidemic—Mandatory Reporting for Glycosylated Hemoglobin Values in New York City," *New England Journal of Medicine*, February 9, 2006.

Steinbrook is a physician and a medical writer for the *New England Journal of Medicine*.

> "Diabetes can lead to serious complications, such as blindness, kidney damage, cardiovascular disease, and lower-limb amputations."

—National Diabetes Information Clearinghouse, "National Diabetes Statistics, 2007." Bethesda, MD: National Institute of Diabetes and Digestive and Kidney Diseases, National Institutes of Health, 2008.

The National Diabetes Information Clearinghouse collects resource information about diabetes for the National Institute of Diabetes and Digestive and Kidney Disorders Reference Collection.

> "I have seen people in their thirties and forties die from overwhelming complications of diabetes. Poorly treated diabetes is like a cancer and can be equally devastating and just as rapid."

—Anne L. Peters, *Conquering Diabetes*. New York: Hudson Street, 2005.

Peters is a professor of medicine and the director of the University of Southern California's clinical diabetes programs. She is the former chairperson of the American Diabetes Association Council on Health Care Delivery and Public Health.

How Serious Is Diabetes?

> "The burden of diabetes is imposed on all sectors of society—higher insurance premiums paid by employees and employers, reduced earnings through productivity loss, and reduced overall quality of life for people with diabetes and their families and friends."

—American Diabetes Association, "Economic Costs of Diabetes in the U.S. in 2007," *Diabetes Care*, March 2008.

The American Diabetes Association funds and advocates for research, publishes scientific findings, advocates for the rights of people with diabetes, and provides information and services to people with diabetes, their families, health-care professionals, and the public.

> "Until we resolve as a nation to make fundamental changes in the healthcare system, people [with diabetes] will die unnecessarily, and doctors, no matter how caring, will not be able to treat everyone who needs their help."

—Francine Ratner Kaufman, *Diabesity*. New York: Bantam, 2006.

Kaufman is the director of the Comprehensive Childhood Diabetes Center and head of the Center for Endocrinology, Diabetes and Metabolism at Children's Hospital in Los Angeles.

> "The increased observation of type 2 diabetes in children is especially alarming—because as younger people develop the disease, the complications, morbidity, and mortality associated with diabetes are all likely to occur earlier."

—Steven Galson, "Childhood Overweight and Type 2 Diabetes: Twin Concerns," Remarks prepared for the plenary address to the CDC Diabetes Translation Conference, Orlando, FL, May 6, 2008.

Galson became acting surgeon general in October 2007.

Facts and Illustrations

How Serious Is Diabetes?

- In 2007, **1.6 million new cases** of diabetes were diagnosed in people aged 20 years or older.

- It is estimated that more than **4,000** new cases of diabetes are diagnosed each day.

- Approximately **23 percent** of Americans over 60 years old have diabetes.

- At least **one-fourth** of American adults are known to have prediabetes.

- Each year approximately **15,000 children** and adolescents are diagnosed with type 1 diabetes.

- Type 2 diabetes, previously considered an adult disease, has increased dramatically in **children and adolescents**.

- **One-third** of U.S. children born in 2000 will develop type 2 diabetes during their lifetime.

- Approximately **one in every five** health-care dollars in the United States is spent caring for someone with diabetes.

- Experts estimate that it costs **$10,000 a year** for a person with diabetes to receive the ongoing medical care they need to keep their blood sugar levels low and under control.

How Serious Is Diabetes?

Number of People with Diabetes Growing

The Centers for Disease Control and Prevention estimates that 23.5 million adults over age 19 had diabetes in 2007 and over twice that many, 57 million adults over age 19, had blood sugar higher than normal. The latter group has prediabetes and is at high risk for developing type 2 diabetes. Studies have shown that losing weight and exercising 30 minutes a day can prevent diabetes among those who have prediabetes. Without preventive action, the number of people with diabetes will continue to grow each year.

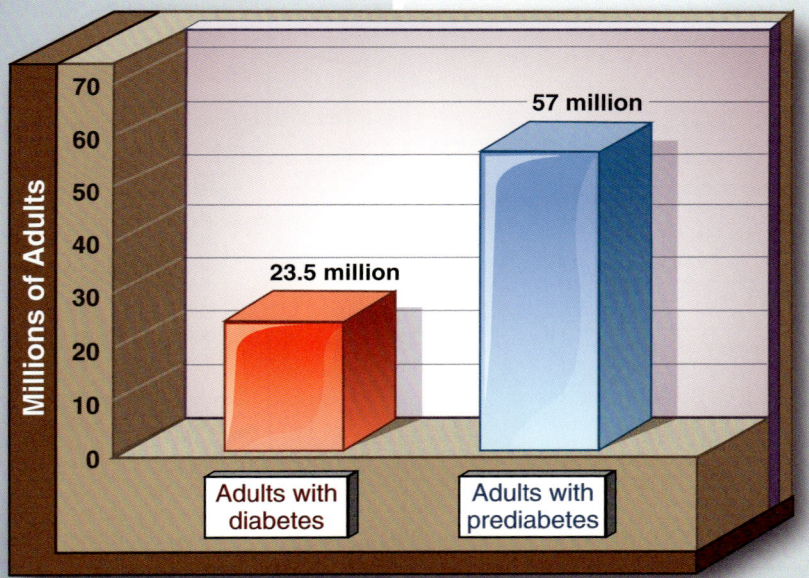

Sources: National Diabetes Information Clearinghouse, "National Diabetes Statistics, 2007," National Institute of Diabetes and Digestive and Kidney Diseases, National Institutes of Health. www.niddk.nih.gov.

- Life expectancy of people with diabetes is **10 to 15 years less** than that of the general U.S. population.

- Men diagnosed with diabetes by age 40 will lose more than **11 years** of life; women diagnosed by age 40 will lose **14 years** of life.

Diabetes

Diabetes Has Many Complications

People with diabetes lack the normal system of checks and balances that keep the body's blood sugar level within a certain range. Without treatment, diabetes kills. Even with treatment, there can be long-term complications of the disease. Over time, excess glucose in the blood puts every organ in the body at risk, causing damage to the eyes, nerves, blood vessels, heart, and kidneys, among other organs. Careful control of blood sugar levels through the use of insulin or oral medications, diet, and exercise helps prevent long-term complications of diabetes, although the longer someone has diabetes, the more likely they are to suffer complications.

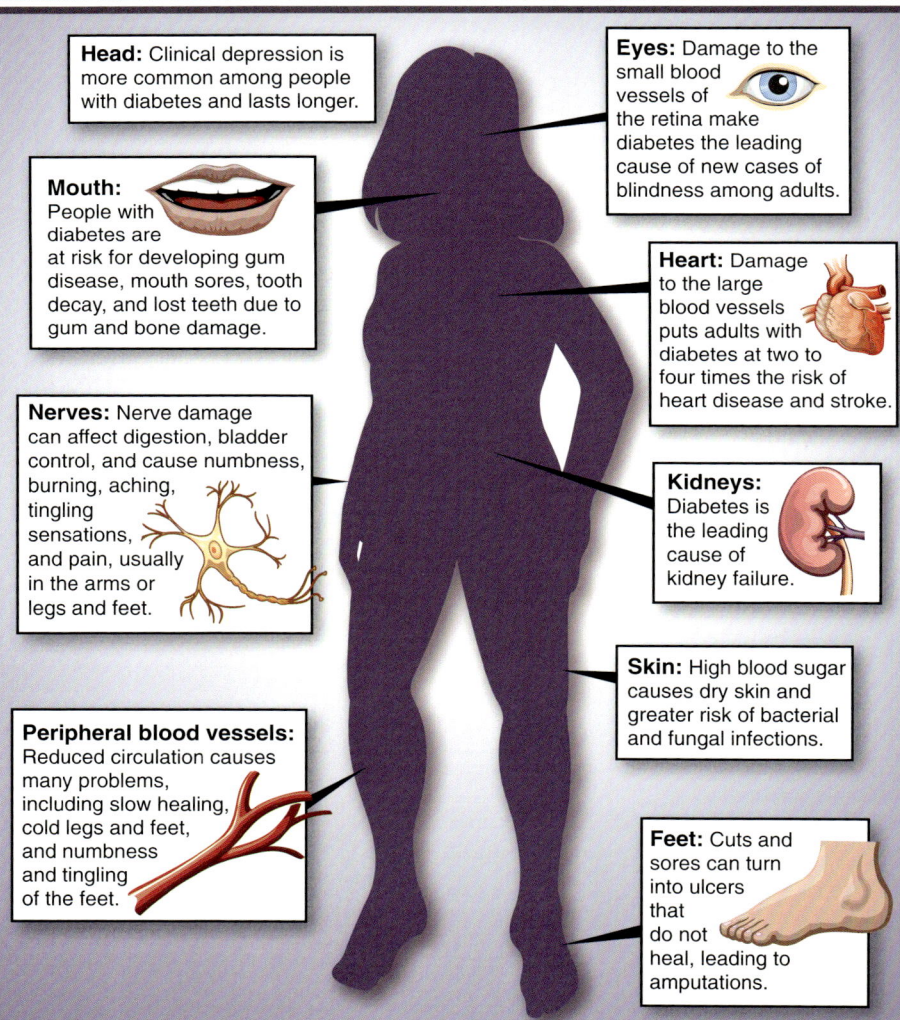

Head: Clinical depression is more common among people with diabetes and lasts longer.

Mouth: People with diabetes are at risk for developing gum disease, mouth sores, tooth decay, and lost teeth due to gum and bone damage.

Nerves: Nerve damage can affect digestion, bladder control, and cause numbness, burning, aching, tingling sensations, and pain, usually in the arms or legs and feet.

Peripheral blood vessels: Reduced circulation causes many problems, including slow healing, cold legs and feet, and numbness and tingling of the feet.

Eyes: Damage to the small blood vessels of the retina make diabetes the leading cause of new cases of blindness among adults.

Heart: Damage to the large blood vessels puts adults with diabetes at two to four times the risk of heart disease and stroke.

Kidneys: Diabetes is the leading cause of kidney failure.

Skin: High blood sugar causes dry skin and greater risk of bacterial and fungal infections.

Feet: Cuts and sores can turn into ulcers that do not heal, leading to amputations.

Sources: Nancy Touchette, *American Diabetes Association Complete Guide to Diabetes*. Alexandria, VA: American Diabetes Association, 2005; American Medical Association, ed. Boyd E. Metzger, *Guide to Living with Diabetes*. Hoboken, NJ: Wiley and Sons, 2006; National Diabetes Information and Digestive and Kidney Diseases, National Institutes of Health, www.niddk.nih.gov; Stephanie A. Eisenstat, David M. Nathan, and Ellen Barlow, *Every Woman's Guide to Diabetes*. Cambridge, MA: Harvard University Press, 2007.

How Serious Is Diabetes?

The Cost of Diabetes

The total estimated cost of diabetes in 2007 was $174 billion, including $116 billion spent on medical care. People with diabetes use more hospital care and visit the emergency room and their doctors' offices more often than people without diabetes. They also spend more time in nursing facilities, have more home visits, and use more medications and medical supplies than those without diabetes. Half the money spent for medical care treating diabetes is spent on hospital stays. Twenty-three percent of the money spent on medical care is used to pay for medications and supplies.

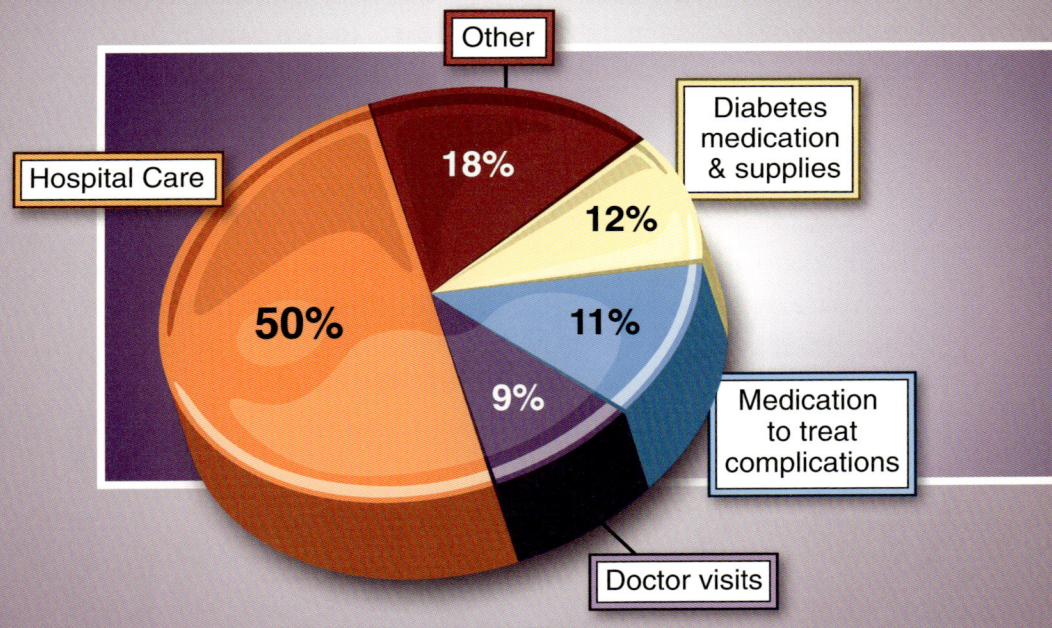

Source: American Diabetes Association, "Economic Costs of Diabetes in the U.S. in 2007," *Diabetes Care*, March 2008.

- Diabetes causes **12,000 to 24,000** new cases of blindness each year.

- Diabetes is the leading cause of kidney failure, accounting for **44 percent** of new cases.

33

What Causes Diabetes?

> **When you visualize the tiny drop of insulin that represents what is missing in your loved one's body, it seems too trivial. Scientists can do so much—how is it they cannot coax the cells to make this tiny drop of protein on demand?**
>
> —Gail O'Keefe, mother of two children with diabetes.

> **Just six months ago, I had to bury another cousin of mine who was in his 50s because of diabetes. And they're getting younger, because of being overweight, not exercising. It's family history for me.**
>
> —Irma Dowden, diagnosed with type 2 diabetes at age 36, now age 42.

Diabetes occurs when a person loses the ability to use glucose, the main sugar that fuels the body. As food goes through the digestive system, mixing with saliva and gastric juices, it is broken down into its components. Carbohydrates, found in grains, fruits, vegetables, dairy products, and sweets, are broken into three main types of sugars: glucose, fructose, and galactose. Of the three, glucose is the main sugar used by the body.

About half the glucose generated by a meal is stored as glycogen in the muscles and liver, to be used later. If the supply of glucose in the blood decreases—say a person exercises and the muscles need more food—the liver releases glucose into the bloodstream to nourish the cells. The supply of glucose in the blood—the blood sugar level—is carefully regulated by

What Causes Diabetes?

the pancreas to ensure that the cells have as much glucose as they need but that excess glucose is not left hanging around in the bloodstream. For a person with diabetes, this system of checks and balances does not work.

Beta Cells and Insulin

The pancreas is a soft, spongy organ shaped a bit like a banana, with a thick end that trails off into a small tail. Located behind the stomach at the level of the navel, the pancreas produces several substances that help the body digest and use food. The bulk of the pancreas produces digestive juices, but scattered throughout the pancreas are clusters of cells, like small islands, called the islets of Langerhans. Within the islets are three types of cells: alpha, beta, and delta cells. All three produce hormones that regulate the body's use of sugar. When blood sugar levels rise, the beta cells release the hormone insulin. Insulin travels through the blood and functions as a "key" to open the doors of the cells and allow glucose to enter. Without insulin to bind to the cell membrane, glucose cannot enter to nourish the cell.

> **Diabetes occurs when a person loses the ability to use glucose, the main sugar that fuels the body.**

People with diabetes either do not produce enough insulin or their cells do not recognize and bind properly to the insulin available. The result is that glucose cannot enter the cells. The cells start to die, and sugar builds up in the blood. The kidneys work to remove the excess sugar, creating the classic symptoms of diabetes: sugar in the urine, frequent urination to remove the sugar, and constant thirst to replace the water being expelled along with the sugar.

Type 1 Diabetes

Type 1 diabetes is usually diagnosed in childhood or adolescence and used to be called "juvenile diabetes" or "insulin-dependent diabetes." Typical onset occurs between ages 8 and 18, although type 1 diabetes can occur at any age. Type 1 diabetes is an autoimmune disease. For some reason the immune system mistakenly identifies the beta cells of the pancreas as foreign cells and attacks and destroys them. The cause

Diabetes

> "Type 1 diabetes is an autoimmune disease. For some reason the immune system mistakenly identifies the beta cells of the pancreas as foreign cells and attacks and destroys them."

of the mistake is not fully known, but experts believe some people are born with a genetic susceptibility that is triggered by something in the environment—perhaps a virus or toxin. Children from families with a strong history of type 1 diabetes or who have a family member with type 1 diabetes are at greater risk, but most of the time there is no known history of type 1 diabetes in the family. Affected children are usually thin to normal weight.

Symptoms of type 1 diabetes come on suddenly and include weight loss, weakness, excessive hunger and thirst, blurred vision, and increased urination. Wess Holston, diagnosed with type 1 diabetes at age 16, lost 27 pounds (12.25kg) in 2 weeks and remembers, "I was real weak and could hardly lift up anything. And I was constantly going to the bathroom."[17]

Destruction of the insulin-producing beta cells of the pancreas leaves the person unable to produce insulin and thus unable to use glucose to power the body. It is impossible to survive without insulin. People with type 1 diabetes must take insulin several times a day, typically by injection, although insulin pumps inserted under the skin are becoming more popular. Insulin cannot be taken orally as a pill because digestive enzymes in the stomach destroy the hormone.

Type 2 Diabetes

Ninety to 95 percent of people with diabetes in the United States have type 2 diabetes. Type 2 diabetes used to be called "non-insulin-dependent diabetes" because people with type 2 diabetes can still produce insulin. For those with type 2 diabetes, the beta cells in the pancreas still work, but either they do not produce enough insulin or the cells in the body have become resistant to insulin's effects. That is, fewer of the receptors on the cell walls recognize and attach to insulin, so less glucose can enter to be used by the cells. Glucose builds up in the blood, triggering the pancreas to produce more insulin. Over time the pancreas gets tired and cannot keep up with the demand for more insulin, and type 2 diabetes develops.

The symptoms of type 2 diabetes come on gradually because the pancreas continues struggling to keep up with the demand for insulin. As long as the pancreas can keep up, the problem remains hidden. Maria Collazo-Clavell, medical instructor at Mayo Medical School, notes, "Lack of symptoms and the slow emergence of the disease are two reasons type 2 diabetes often goes undetected for years."[18] When symptoms do develop, they vary. However, most people experience excessive thirst and the need to urinate frequently. Other symptoms include extreme hunger, fatigue, unusual weight loss, blurred vision, frequent infections, or sores that are slow to heal.

People with type 2 diabetes are almost always overweight. Type 2 diabetes also tends to run in families. However, as Boyd E. Metzger of the American Medical Association notes, "Although there is a genetic component in type 2 diabetes, it does not mean type 2 diabetes is an inherited disorder."[19] Type 2 diabetes seems to be caused by the interaction of several genes that make a person susceptible to diabetes and lifestyle and environmental factors. Key among the lifestyle factors that contribute to diabetes are obesity and lack of exercise. Smoking, stress, and lack of sleep can also increase insulin resistance, putting a person at risk of diabetes.

> **For those with type 2 diabetes, the beta cells in the pancreas still work, but they either do not produce enough insulin or the cells in the body have become resistant to insulin's effects.**

The lifestyle factors that increase the risk for type 2 diabetes also contribute to a type of diabetes recently identified as type 1.5 diabetes. This new type of diabetes is "the consequence of type 1 diabetes in a progressively obese population,"[20] says Philip Zeitler, associate professor of pediatrics at the University of Colorado Health Sciences Center in Denver. People with type 1.5 diabetes essentially have double diabetes. They have

Diabetes

lost their ability to produce insulin due to type 1 diabetes and have developed a resistance to insulin, which is associated with type 2 diabetes. The 2 conditions together make the disease even harder to manage.

Gestational Diabetes

Gestational diabetes develops during pregnancy among 2 to 5 percent of pregnant women. The growing baby and the hormones produced increase the body's demand for insulin. If the beta cells of the pancreas cannot keep up, the pregnant woman develops gestational diabetes.

> **People with type 1.5 diabetes have double diabetes. They have lost their ability to produce insulin due to type 1 diabetes and have developed resistance to insulin, which is associated with type 2 diabetes.**

Most women with gestational diabetes return to having normal blood sugar levels after they give birth, but they have a 40 to 60 percent chance of developing type 2 diabetes within the next 5 to 10 years. Children of mothers who had gestational diabetes are also at greater risk of developing type 2 diabetes later in life, especially if the mother's blood sugar level was poorly controlled. These children are more likely to be overweight and have high blood pressure than are children whose mothers maintained blood sugar levels within normal range. If gestational diabetes goes undiagnosed and untreated, the baby is likely to be large in size, stillborn, or suffer newborn complications such as jaundice.

Prediabetes

Diabetes experts have identified a stage they call prediabetes. This occurs when blood sugar levels are higher than normal, but not high enough for the person to be diagnosed with diabetes. It is estimated that 57 million adults in the United States had prediabetes in 2007. People with prediabetes are at high risk for developing type 2 diabetes and heart disease, even though they have no symptoms other than an elevated blood sugar level on a screening test.

Studies have shown that people with prediabetes can delay or prevent the onset of type 2 diabetes by making lifestyle changes. The Diabetes Prevention Program, a national clinical trial, found that type 2 diabetes could be prevented or delayed by doing 30 minutes of moderate exercise a day in combination with a 5 to 7 percent loss in body weight. That's the equivalent of a person who weighs 175 pounds (79.4kg) losing about 9 to 12 pounds (4 to 5.4kg).

Metabolic Syndrome

According to Francine Ratner Kaufman, past president of the American Diabetes Association, "Approximately one-third of obese adults, and perhaps as many overweight teenagers, have metabolic syndrome."[21] Also called "syndrome X" or "insulin resistance syndrome," metabolic syndrome is a cluster of risk factors for diabetes and heart disease. The risk factors include higher-than-normal blood sugar levels, a large waist circumference, high blood pressure, high triglycerides (a form of fat carried in the blood), and low levels of high-density lipoproteins—a type of cholesterol that protects against heart disease. People with metabolic syndrome have a characteristic apple shape, with excess weight around their middle. The more overweight they are, the greater the risk for heart disease and diabetes.

Metabolic syndrome is largely caused by chemical signals from fat cells. These signals trigger inflammation similar to that experienced when nasal passages swell from a cold or to the swelling, heat, and soreness around a cut. Normally, inflammation helps us heal, but too much fat can cause chronic inflammation throughout the body, including inflammation of the blood vessels. The inflamed blood vessels become narrower, restricting blood flow. If there are cholesterol deposits along the blood vessel walls, they can distort the walls of the blood vessels or break off and form blood clots that can cause a stroke or heart attack. The inflammation caused by excess fat seems to

> **Studies have shown that people with prediabetes can delay or prevent the onset of type 2 diabetes by making lifestyle changes.**

be the link between obesity, diabetes, and heart disease that occurs with metabolic syndrome.

Who Is at Risk?

Both type 1 and type 2 diabetes appear to be triggered by something in the environment that affects people with a genetic predisposition for the disease. However the precise genetics and environmental causes are still being explored. For example, young non-Hispanic white children and adolescents are at highest risk of getting type 1 diabetes but no one knows why. If one identical twin gets type 1 diabetes, there is only a 40 percent chance the other twin will develop type 1 diabetes in his or her lifetime. In addition, the risk for type 1 diabetes is only 1 to 6 percent greater for someone who has a parent or sibling with the disease.

Unlike type 1 diabetes, type 2 tends to run in families. A person with one parent or a sibling who has type 2 diabetes has a 14 to 25 percent greater chance of getting type 2 diabetes than someone without a close relative with the disease. If both parents have type 2 diabetes, the risk goes up to 75 percent. But even without a family history, people who weigh 20 percent or more above the ideal weight for their height and who do not exercise are at risk for type 2 diabetes.

Unlike type 1 diabetes, where young whites are at greatest risk, those most at risk in the United States for type 2 diabetes are Native Americans, African Americans, Mexican Americans, Puerto Ricans, Pacific Islanders, and Asian Americans. The theory is that these populations have a "thrifty gene" that enhances their ability to survive when food is in short supply. It is an adaptive response that has been useful for much of human history and has allowed people to survive famine and long winters. But when food is readily available and the need for physical labor is decreased, people with the thrifty gene can gain weight rapidly, becoming obese and at risk for type 2 diabetes.

The link between genetic and environmental factors is still being explored, and scientists continue to study why certain ethnic groups are at greater risk for one type of diabetes than another. Through greater understanding of the disease process, scientists may be able to find a cure for diabetes.

Primary Source Quotes*

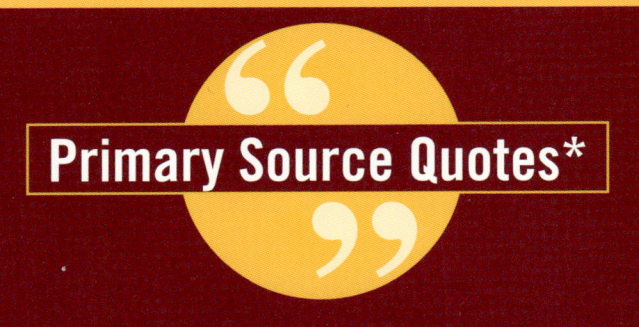

What Causes Diabetes?

66 While [type 1 and type 2] diabetes have clear medical differences, they are both characterized by the loss of beta cells. Type 2 patients experience the loss more gradually, but inexorably, and they will eventually need insulin to survive, just like their type 1 counterparts. 99

—James S. Hirsch. *Cheating Destiny: Living with Diabetes.* Boston: Houghton Mifflin, 2006.

Hirsch is a former reporter for the *New York Times* and the *Wall Street Journal*, who was diagnosed with type 1 diabetes at age 15 and who has a son and brother who also have type 1 diabetes.

66 It is hard to detect type 2 diabetes in children because it can go undiagnosed for a long time; because children may have no symptoms or mild symptoms; and because blood tests are needed for diagnosis. 99

—National Center for Chronic Disease Prevention and Health Promotion, Centers for Disease Control and Prevention, "Diabetes Projects," September 30, 2008. www.cdc.gov.

The National Center for Chronic Disease and Prevention and Health Promotion conducts studies to better understand the causes of chronic diseases. It is part of the Centers for Disease Control and Prevention.

* Editor's Note: While the definition of a primary source can be narrowly or broadly defined, for the purposes of Compact Research, a primary source consists of: 1) results of original research presented by an organization or researcher; 2) eyewitness accounts of events, personal experience, or work experience; 3) first-person editorials offering pundits' opinions; 4) government officials presenting political plans and/or policies; 5) representatives of organizations presenting testimony or policy.

Diabetes

> "I consider myself lucky. I had symptoms that brought me to the doctor, whereas for many people (type 2) diabetes is a silent killer."

—Stephanie A. Eisenstat, quoted in Stephanie A. Eisenstat, David M. Nathan, and Ellen Barlow, *Every Woman's Guide to Diabetes*. Cambridge, MA: Harvard University Press, 2007.

Eisenstat is an internist with Women's Health Associates at Massachusetts General Hospital and an assistant professor of medicine and scholar at the Academy at Harvard Medical School.

> "I was diagnosed with diabetes in 1997 at age 27. I didn't know anyone else my age with diabetes, and I considered myself a pretty healthy person. That vision of myself probably delayed diagnosis: I just kept brushing off the symptoms as 'stress.'"

—Heather Nielsen Clute, "The Ride of a Lifetime: Supporting Diabetes Education," *MyTCOYD*, first quarter, 2008.

Clute, now 38, uses insulin to manage her diabetes. She lives in Europe, competes in triathlons, and has a family.

> "Obesity is one of the risk factors for developing type 2 diabetes. In the United States, there are widespread and growing epidemics of both obesity and diabetes in adults and children."

—Richard S. Beaser and Amy P. Campbell, *The Joslin Guide to Diabetes*. New York: Fireside, 2005.

Beaser is the medical executive director of professional education at the Joslin Diabetes Center in Boston and an associate clinical professor at the Harvard Medical School. Campbell is a registered dietitian and education program manager of the Disease Management Department at the Joslin Diabetes Center.

What Causes Diabetes?

❝Simply put, we're moving our bodies less, eating more, and eating more of the wrong foods.❞

—David M. Nathan and Linda M. Delahanty, *Beating Diabetes: The First Complete Program Clinically Proven to Dramatically Improve Your Glucose Tolerance.* New York: McGraw-Hill, 2005.

Nathan is a professor of medicine at Harvard Medical School and the director of the Diabetes Center at Massachusetts General Hospital. Delahanty is chief dietitian and director of Nutrition and Behavioral Research at the Diabetes Center at Massachusetts General Hospital.

❝[Type 2 diabetes] usually begins as insulin resistance, a disorder in which the cells do not use insulin properly. As the need for insulin rises, the pancreas gradually loses its ability to produce it.❞

—National Diabetes Information Clearinghouse, "National Diabetes Statistics, 2007." Bethesda, MD: National Institute of Diabetes and Digestive and Kidney Diseases, National Institutes of Health, 2008.

The National Diabetes Information Clearinghouse collects resource information about diabetes for the National Institute of Diabetes and Digestive and Kidney Disorders Reference Collection.

❝Families like [my patient's] are common now: a massively obese child and that youngster's equally heavy relatives, some of whom—even men and women in their twenties, thirties, or forties—already show the terrible long-term effects of diabetes.❞

—Francine Ratner Kaufman, *Diabesity.* New York: Bantam, 2006.

Kaufman is the director of the Comprehensive Childhood Diabetes Center and head of the Center for Endocrinology, Diabetes and Metabolism at Children's Hospital in Los Angeles and a past president of the American Diabetes Association.

Facts and Illustrations

What Causes Diabetes?

- Type 1 diabetes develops when the **pancreas** makes little if any insulin.

- In type 1 diabetes the beta cells of the pancreas are **destroyed**, leaving the body unable to produce insulin.

- Type 1 diabetes can occur at any age, but most commonly occurs in **children and adolesents**.

- In adults type 1 diabetes accounts for **5 to 10 percent** of all diagnosed cases of diabetes.

- Type 2 diabetes is a problem of both **insulin resistance** and **insulin deficiency**.

- Type 2 diabetes remains **extremely rare** among children under 10 years old.

- Among white youths aged **10 to 19 years**, new cases of type 1 diabetes exceed new cases of type 2 diabetes. The opposite is true for Asian, Pacific Islander, and American Indian youth.

- In adults type 2 diabetes accounts for **90 to 95 percent** of all diagnosed cases of diabetes.

What Causes Diabetes?

Race and Diabetes

Diabetes is more common in some racial or ethnic groups than others. Type 1 diabetes is most common in people of non-Hispanic, northern European descent, followed by African Americans and Hispanic Americans. It is relatively rare in people of Asian descent. The group at greatest risk of developing type 2 diabetes is African Americans.

Race/ethnicity	Total U.S. population	With diagnosed diabetes		With undiagnosed diabetes		Total with diabetes*	
	In thousands						
African American	37,002	2,775	7.5%	699	1.9%	3,474	9.4%
Non-Hispanic white	199,091	11,403	5.7%	4,520	2.3%	15,923	8.0%
Hispanic	45,541	2,231	4.9%	1,104	2.4%	3,335	7.3%
Non-Hispanic other	20,101	1,076	5.4%	317	1.6%	1,393	6.9%
Total population*	301,765	17,485	5.8%	6,640	2.2%	24,125	8.0%

*Numbers do not necessarily sum to totals because of rounding.
Source: CDC, *Diabetes Care*, March 2008. www.cdc.gov.

- A weight gain of **11 to 18 pounds** (5 to 8.2kg) increases a person's risk of developing type 2 diabetes to twice that of individuals who have not gained weight.

- **Eighty to 90 percent** of people with type 2 diabetes are overweight or obese.

- In the national Diabetes Prevention Program study conducted from 1997 to 2001 and still considered an important resource for diabetes prevention statistics, **weight loss** was the main predictor of reduced risk for diabetes.

Diabetes

The Pancreas and Diabetes

The pancreas is located behind the stomach at the level of the navel and produces a number of substances that are used for digestion. Most of the pancreas consists of acinar cells that produce digestive juices, which flow through ducts into the small intestine. Scattered throughout the acinar cells are islands of cells of a different type, called the islets of Langerhans. The islets of Langerhans contain alpha, beta, and delta cells, all of which produce hormones that regulate the body's use of sugar. Type 1 diabetes occurs when the beta cells die and can no longer produce the hormone insulin. Type 2 diabetes occurs when the beta cells cannot keep up with the body's demand for insulin.

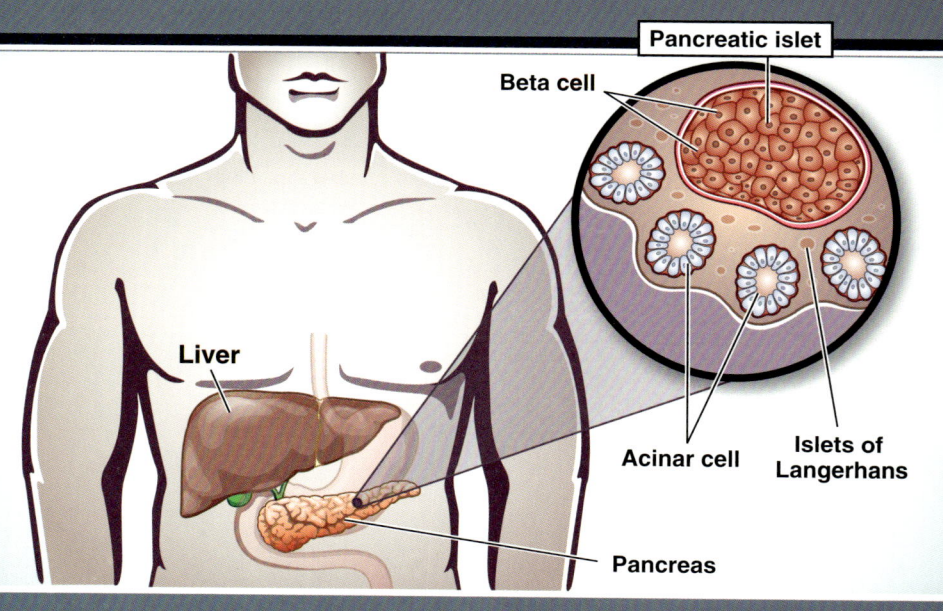

Sources: Melvin R. Hayden, "Islet Amyloid, Metabolic Syndrome, and the Natural Progressive History of Type 2 Diabetes Mellitus," *Journal of the Pancreas*, September 2002; National Diabetes Information Clearinghouse, "Pancreatic Islet Transplant," National Diabetes Statistics, 2007," National Institute of Diabetes and Digestive and Kidney Diseases, National Institutes of Health, www.niddk.nih.gov; Rosemary Walker and Jill Rodgers in association with the American Diabetes Association, *Diabetes: A Practical Guide to Managing Your Health*. New York: Dorling Kindersley, 2005.

- Women who have had gestational diabetes have a **40 to 60 percent** chance of developing diabetes in the ensuing 5 to 10 years.

What Causes Diabetes?

Characteristics of Type 1 and Type 2 Diabetes

Although in both type 1 and type 2 diabetes the body lacks sufficient insulin, they are separate conditions due to different causes. This table places the key characteristics of each disease side-by-side for comparison.

	Type 1 Diabetes	Type 2 Diabetes
Age of Onset	Most frequently diagnosed in children and adolescents. Rarely develops after age 40	Most frequently diagnosed in people over 40 years old, although it is becoming more common among young adults and teens
Body Weight	Typically thin to normal weight	Typically overweight
Type of Onset	Rapid onset. Diagnosed typically within days or weeks of the development of symptoms	Slow onset with symptoms occurring gradually over months or years. Classic symptoms may not be present. Diagnosis may not occur for years after the condition begins
Effect	The body produces no insulin, because the beta cells have been destroyed	Insulin is still produced, but the body is resistant to its action. Over time, insulin production decreases
Cause	Autoimmune reaction destroys the beta cells of the pancreas	Not well understood. Appears to be a combination of genetics, lifestyle, insulin resistance, and insufficient production of insulin
Symptoms	Frequent urination, excessive thirst, weight loss, and fatigue that come on quickly and are severe	Frequent urination and excessive thirst. Weight loss, fatigue, and blurred vision. May come on gradually
Treatment	Must take insulin several times a day	Can use oral medication or insulin. Some can reverse the disease by weight loss, diet, and exercise
Risk Factors	Slightly increased risk if another family member has disease	Over age 45, overweight, and inactive. Increased risk by 14 percent for each family member with type 2 diabetes. Increased risk if Native American, African American, Hispanic, Pacific Islander, or Asian American
Cure	No known cure	No known cure

Sources: National Diabetes Information Clearinghouse, "Diagnosis of Diabetes," National Institute of Diabetes and Digestive and Kidney Diseases, National Institutes of Health. www.niddk.nih.gov; Christopher D. Suadek, Richard R. Rubin, and Cynthia S. Shump, *The Johns Hopkins Guide to Diabetes for Today and Tomorrow*. Baltimore: Johns Hopkins University Press, 1997; Rosemary Walker and Jill Rodgers in association with the American Diabetes Association, *Diabetes: A Practical Guide to Managing Your Health*. New York: Dorling Kindersley, 2004; Janice M. Yuwiler, *Great Medical Discoveries: Insulin*. Detroit: Lucent, 2005.

How Is Diabetes Treated?

“The burdens [of type 1 and type 2 diabetes] are also similar, requiring a daily juggle of diet, exercise, and medication to maintain a normal blood sugar—which is to say, an unusual amount of self-discipline and personal initiative.”

—James S. Hirsch, diagnosed with diabetes at age 15 and author of *Cheating Destiny: Living with Diabetes.*

“I know now that I also want the [insulin] pump because then you can eat all the time and you don't need to wake up early to do your blood glucose and injection.”

—Douglas, a 12-year-old with type 1 diabetes.

The first step toward treating diabetes is diagnosis. Almost 25 percent of Americans with diabetes do not know they have the disease, yet it could be identified via a blood test. A person is diagnosed with diabetes when blood drawn in the morning after an overnight fast shows an elevated blood sugar level of 126 milligrams per deciliter (mg/dl) or more. (Normal blood sugar levels range from 70 to 100 mg/dl.) Those with fasting blood sugar levels of 100–125 mg/dl have prediabetes. Their blood sugar levels are higher than normal, but not high enough to have diabetes, although they are at high risk for getting diabetes within the next 10 years.

Blood sugar levels vary throughout the day and are typically highest after eating and lowest in the morning after an overnight fast. Exercise also lowers blood sugar levels as the muscles take in glucose for energy. Normally the pancreas and liver form a feedback loop based on the amount of glucose in the blood. The result is a normal blood sugar level in the range of 70 to 100 mg/dl. Even after eating, the blood sugar level will rarely rise above 180 mg/dl.

For a person with diabetes, the feedback loop does not work. People with diabetes need to balance food intake and their physical activity with dosages of insulin or other medications. As Kaufman tells her patients, "You must become your own pancreas."[22]

The importance of maintaining near-to-normal blood sugar levels was proved by the Diabetes Control and Complications Trial. Conducted by 29 medical centers in the United States and Canada from 1983 to 1989, the study found participants who kept their blood sugar levels close to normal cut their risk of kidney disease by 50 percent, their risk of nerve damage by 60 percent, and their risk of blindness by 76 percent. As a result, people with diabetes now strive to maintain blood sugar levels between 70 and 90 mg/dl.

Types of Insulin

All people with type 1 diabetes, and eventually many with type 2 diabetes, must take insulin to replace the insulin their pancreases no longer produce. The trick is to balance the amount of insulin taken so that more insulin is available during mealtimes and less at night, when blood sugar levels fall. There are a variety of insulins on the market; some work quickly but do not last long while others take several hours to start working but the effects last longer. The type of insulin needed depends on an individual's unique activity and eating habits.

Taking Insulin

For decades the only way to take insulin was via injection, because digestive juices in the stomach destroy insulin taken in pill form. Today, small syringes with thin needles make injections nearly painless. Insulin pen injectors, that look like a cartridge pen and can store and deliver a dose of insulin, make insulin injection easier and more discreet. Insulin infusers inserted under the skin of the abdomen or hip allow daily insulin to be injected into the infuser's flexible, hollow tube, or catheter, instead of directly through the skin. And insulin pumps, small devices that are connected to an infusion set and worn like a pager, can store and deliver insulin via a catheter as programmed by the user, making frequent delivery of insulin easier.

Recently, alternate methods of taking insulin have come on the market. Insulin jet injectors send a fine spray of insulin through the skin using pressurized air. The first form of inhaled insulin was approved for use in 2006. And work is under way to develop an insulin patch, along the lines of the nicotine patch. Although promising, these techniques may not completely replace the need to inject insulin. An injection of insulin may still be needed to maintain a baseline level of insulin or to obtain a large dose of insulin at mealtime.

Oral Medications

Not all people with diabetes take insulin injections. Most of those with type 2 diabetes begin by taking oral medications designed either to increase the pancreas's production of insulin or to reduce the impact of the body's resistance to insulin. Two classes of drugs, sulfonylureas and meglitinides, cause the pancreas to produce more insulin. Another group, the biguanides, improve the body's response to insulin by reducing the amount of glucose released by the liver between meals, thus reducing the amount of insulin needed. The alpha-glucosidase inhibitors slow down digestion of carbohydrates into sugars and prevent sugar products from being absorbed by the intestine. Both actions slow the normal rise of blood sugar after a meal, which gives the available insulin more time to do its job. Finally, the thiazolidinediones work to enhance the natural action of insulin in the body by making the cell walls more sensitive to insulin and increasing the liver's ability to store glucose.

> **People with diabetes need to balance food intake and their physical activity with dosages of insulin or other medications.**

Oral medications are not a cure and may cause side effects of their own. A person can develop tolerance to the medication so that it stops working over time, and there is always the risk of hypoglycemia should the medication build up and cause a dangerously low blood sugar level. Hypoglycemia occurs when too much insulin moves glucose into the cells and the blood

How Is Diabetes Treated?

sugar level drops. In addition there is a tendency to believe taking medication controls the disease. Richard S. Beaser and Joan V.C. Hill, authors of *The Joslin Guide to Diabetes*, note, "People often make the mistake of abandoning their meal

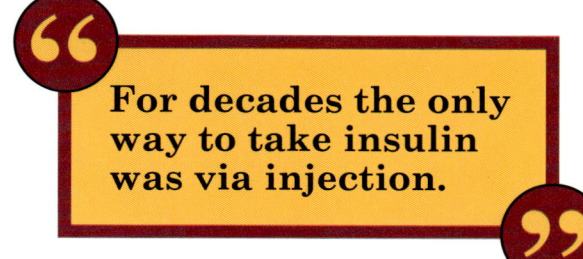

> "For decades the only way to take insulin was via injection."

plan or exercise program, believing the tablets alone will handle their diabetes. But as effective as these pills may be, they can't take care of your diabetes themselves."[23]

Diet and Exercise

People with diabetes must pay more attention to the amount and type of food they eat and when they consume it than those without diabetes. James S. Hirsch, a diabetic since the age of 15, imagines insulin and food like two

> armies in the night battling inside a diabetic's body. Survival requires a balance of forces. If one becomes too strong (for example, if you overeat), then reinforcements are needed (you require more insulin). And if one army has retreated entirely (you skip several shots or meals), the remaining brigade of rampaging food or unchecked insulin unleashes its destructive force on the body itself, causing ketoacidosis or hypoglycemic coma.[24]

There is no single diabetes diet. For example, someone overweight with type 2 diabetes may need to eat a different ratio of carbohydrate to protein than a thin person with type 1 diabetes who is at risk for kidney disease. In general people with type 1 diabetes and those with type 2 diabetes who take insulin use one of several different methods for tracking the food they eat. Diabetic exchange lists help people maintain a proper balance of carbohydrates, fats and proteins. Carbohydrate counting tracks the number of carbohydrates consumed each day. And the glycemic index is a way to track how quickly different types of carbohydrates increase blood sugar. A heart-healthy diet with most carbohydrates coming from vegetables, fruits, beans and whole grains is commonly recommended, but because everyone is different, experts suggest a nutritionist familiar with diabetes be consulted.

Given the link between obesity and diabetes, reaching and maintaining a healthy weight is a key goal for people with type 2 diabetes. Weight loss increases the body's sensitivity to insulin, allowing the body to lower blood sugar levels naturally by using the available insulin produced by the pancreas. Studies comparing most of the popular diets, including high-carbohydrate/high fiber diets, low-fat diets, and diets designed to manage weight showed that any healthy diet that helps someone to lose weight and keep it off will help treat diabetes. Experts are divided regarding the amount and type of carbohydrates that should be eaten, but all agree that processed foods high in fat and sugar pose a risk for people with type 2 diabetes.

> **Controlling blood sugar levels is not easy.**

Physical activity also plays an essential role in controlling type 2 diabetes. According to Boyd E. Metzger, "Regular exercise helps stabilize blood glucose levels by improving the body's use of insulin and by burning extra body fat, which improves the cells' sensitivity to insulin."[25] On the advice of her doctor, Erendira, a young woman with diabetes, started walking every day. At the end of the month she told her doctor, "I haven't had sugars so close to normal since I first got diabetes. I'm pretty amazed at what this walking has done."[26]

Controlling Blood Sugar

Controlling blood sugar levels is not easy. Yet David G. Orloff, former director of the Division of Metabolism and Endocrinology Products at the U.S. Food and Drug Administration, reflects the general consensus in the field when he states, "Daily monitoring and careful control of blood sugar levels are the most important steps people with diabetes can take."[27] A 30-year study of 4,400 people with diabetes found that those who kept their blood sugar levels below 300 mg/dl had 3 times fewer complications after 15 years than those with higher blood sugar levels. The results were even better for those with better control, with 5 to 20 times fewer complications among those with blood sugar levels below 250 mg/dl. Those below 120 mg/dl had almost no risk of complications at all.

How Is Diabetes Treated?

Diabetes Burnout

Tight control of blood sugar means injecting insulin or taking oral medication every day at the right time, in the right amount, and eating and exercising to match the level of medication taken. It necessitates pricking a finger multiple times a day to test blood sugar levels and then making decisions about eating, exercising, or taking more insulin based on the results. It may seem like an easy thing to do, but it is not. An American Diabetes Association study found that 21 percent of adults with type 1 diabetes have never checked their blood sugar level; 41 percent of type 2 diabetics who use insulin do not monitor their blood sugar level; and of those with type 2 diabetes who are not taking insulin, 76 percent never check their blood sugar levels. Of those who do check, many do not check as frequently as they should.

Diet and exercise are equally hard to maintain for many. In a study conducted at the Joslin Diabetes Center and two large clinics in California, 22 percent of patients reported knowing that they should follow a certain meal plan but found it was usually impossible to do so, and 37 to 43 percent never exercised.

> **Tight control of blood sugar means injecting insulin or taking oral medication every day at the right time, in the right amount, and eating and exercising to match the level of medication taken.**

Polonsky notes: "Burnout is what happens when you feel overwhelmed by diabetes and by the frustrating burden of diabetes self-care. People who are burned out realize that good diabetes care is important for their health, but they just don't have the motivation to do it. At a fundamental level, they are at war with their diabetes—and they are losing."[28]

Despite the threat of diabetes burnout, many people with diabetes juggle insulin, oral medications, food intake, and exercise in response to their blood sugar levels, refusing to let diabetes set limits on what they can do. Gary Hall Jr., an Olympic gold medalist, is but one example. In 1999 Hall had four Olympic swimming medals and was training for yet another Olympics when he was diagnosed with type 1 diabetes. Working carefully to monitor and control his blood sugar levels, Hall went on to compete in 2 more Olympic Games. In 2004, at the Summer Olympics, Hall became one of the most decorated athletes in Olympic history.

Hall is not alone. Actresses Halle Berry and Mary Tyler Moore, musicians B.B. King, Randy Jackson, and Nick Jonas, teachers, lawyers, construction workers, and others in all walks of life work daily to manage their diabetes. Dr. Günter Spiro, a pioneer on the impact of diabetes on kidney failure, and a diabetic himself, says, "I think it takes courage to take care of diabetes. It's much easier to let it go."[29] Despite the temptation to eat whenever and whatever they choose and to be free of the restrictions imposed by diabetes, many Americans have had the courage to manage their diabetes and by doing so have warded off diabetes' complications.

Primary Source Quotes*

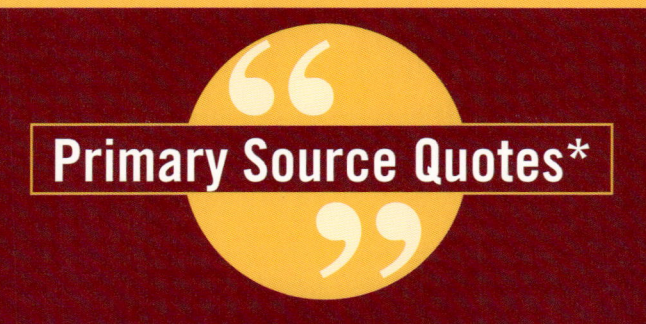

How Is Diabetes Treated?

66 Some diseases are worse than diabetes. But none requires such a complex balancing act, where patients must do so much themselves. 99

—Francine Ratner Kaufman, *Diabesity.* New York: Bantam, 2006.

Kaufman is the director of the Comprehensive Childhood Diabetes Center and head of the Center for Endocrinology, Diabetes, and Metabolism at Children's Hospital in Los Angeles and a past president of the American Diabetes Association.

66 As diabetics we really should consider ourselves lucky that our disease does not explicitly limit our ability to explore and engage with the world and its people. Let us also not forget that if we maintain good glycemic control, even in our elder days, we can find many years of active travel [life] ahead. 99

—Adam M. Levbarg, "Seven Months of Travel in Six Remote Asian Countries by One Type 1 Diabetic (That's Me!)" *MyTCOYD*, third quarter, 2008.

Levbarg spent seven months in Asia using an insulin pump and carrying his insulin and all diabetes-related supplies.

* Editor's Note: While the definition of a primary source can be narrowly or broadly defined, for the purposes of Compact Research, a primary source consists of: 1) results of original research presented by an organization or researcher; 2) eyewitness accounts of events, personal experience, or work experience; 3) first-person editorials offering pundits' opinions; 4) government officials presenting political plans and/or policies; 5) representatives of organizations presenting testimony or policy.

Diabetes

> **I'd take the [insulin] injection before bed, and then I'd awake to paramedics at my side. . . . Then I was affected by the other side of diabetes: high blood sugars. I slipped into near fatal bouts of ketoacidosis.**
>
> —Katherine Marple, "Living with Diabetes: Diabetes Doesn't Define Me," *Diabetes Health*, April 1, 2009. www.diabeteshealth.com.

Marple was diagnosed with type 1 diabetes as a teenager and has struggled to control her blood sugar level, switching between medications numerous times. She now uses an insulin pump.

> **There is a serious lack of two-way communication between providers and patients, and a misunderstanding by the majority of providers about what it is like to live with diabetes on a day-to-day basis.**
>
> —Steven V. Edelman, "Making the Connection: Closing the Delicate Loop Between Professional and Patient Education," *MyTCOYD*, second quarter, 2008.

Edelman is a professor of medicine at the University of California, San Diego. He is also founder and director of the national organization Taking Control of Your Diabetes, which assists patients with managing their diabetes.

> **I am aware of [my diabetes] when I am driving. I am aware of it when I am playing with my kids. And then I have to remember to take insulin before I eat.**
>
> —Julie Ann Ressler, "Diabetes with No Finger Pricks," CBS News, August 7, 2008. www.cbsnews.com.

Ressler has type 1 diabetes, works as a physician, and is the mother of two children. She carries her blood glucose meter with her everywhere. She is also participating in a study at the City of Hope Hospital in Los Angeles to help with the development of an artificial pancreas.

How Is Diabetes Treated?

❝Like many diseases, diabetes is caused by our genes and our personal environment, which is created by our lifestyle. We cannot yet modify our genes, but we can modify our lifestyle.❞

—David M. Nathan and Linda M. Delahanty, *Beating Diabetes: The First Complete Program Clinically Proven to Dramatically Improve Your Glucose Tolerance.* New York: McGraw-Hill, 2005.

Nathan is a professor of medicine at Harvard Medical School and the director of the Diabetes Center at Massachusetts General Hospital. Delahanty is chief dietitian and director of nutrition and behavioral research at the Diabetes Center at Massachusetts General Hospital.

❝Reaching and maintaining a healthy weight is an essential goal for people with type 2 diabetes. Weight loss improves insulin sensitivity, enabling the insulin in your body to more easily lower blood sugar naturally.❞

—Boyd E. Metzger, ed., *American Medical Association Guide to Living with Diabetes.* Hoboken, NJ: Wiley, 2006.

Metzger is the Tom D. Spies Professor of Metabolism and Nutrition in the Division of Endocrinology, Metabolism and Molecular Medicine at Northwestern University Feinberg School of Medicine and editor for the American Medical Association.

❝We diabetics are abundantly human. We miss, forget, foul up, flake on our diabetes regimen, or just don't do enough to take care of ourselves. Frequently our blood glucose simply doesn't cooperate!❞

—Andrew Young, "Mind over Mellitus: Diabetes—a Short Cut to Greatness?" *MyTCOYD*, second quarter, 2008.

Young is the editor of *Mind over Mellitus*, a biweekly newsletter focusing on success with diabetes and life through personal motivation and self-discipline.

Diabetes

❝ No matter how much I weighed and measured and calculated how much insulin I needed . . . my blood glucose was still too high. . . . When [getting a continuous glucose monitor] made it possible for me to control my blood glucose levels, it made me want to maintain that control. ❞

—Jan Chait, "Trying to Control the Uncontrollable," Diabetes Self Management, November, 7, 2006. www.diabetesselfmanagement.com.

Chait has type 2 diabetes and switched from oral medications to insulin to gain better control of her blood sugar levels.

❝ Diabetes also dramatizes the growing divide between the haves and have-nots in medical care. What is emerging is an elite corps of diabetics—highly motivated, educated, and financially secure—who are flourishing . . . compared to the nearly 90 percent who fail to meet basic goals for blood glucose. ❞

—James S. Hirsch, *Cheating Destiny: Living with Diabetes*. Boston: Houghton Mifflin, 2006.

Hirsch is a former reporter for the *New York Times* and the *Wall Street Journal* who was diagnosed with type 1 diabetes at age 15 and has a son and brother who also have type 1 diabetes.

Facts and Illustrations

How Is Diabetes Treated?

- More than **14,000** heart attacks, strokes, and amputations could be prevented each year through better diabetes management.

- Diabetes requires active participation and **self-management** by the patient and also a **knowledgeable and empathetic doctor**.

- According to the National Committee for Quality Assurance, as much as **$1.3 billion** a year in hospital costs could be saved if health-care monitoring for blood sugar levels were improved.

- In 2007, **12.5 million** sick days could have been avoided with better health care for diabetes.

- Monitoring **blood sugar levels** helps people with diabetes manage the disease and avoid complications.

- In the Diabetes Control and Complications Trial, participants who kept their blood sugar levels close to normal reduced their risk of **kidney disease**, **nerve damage**, and **blindness**.

- The percentage of U.S. adults with diabetes meeting recommended goals for blood sugar level increased from 34 percent in 1999 to **56 percent** in 2000.

- In a nationwide survey, **76 percent** of people with type 2 diabetes who used oral medications never checked their blood sugar level; **21 percent** of patients with type 1 diabetes never checked their blood sugar level.

59

Diabetes

Diabetes Food Pyramid

The American Diabetes Association and the American Dietetic Association have developed a food pyramid to help people better manage diabetes on a daily basis. The diabetes food pyramid highlights groups of foods based on their carbohydrate and protein content because these foods affect blood glucose levels and thus are of most concern to people with diabetes.

Fats:
A serving of fat can be: 1/8 avocado
1 Tbsp. cream cheese or salad dressing
1 tsp. butter, margarine, oil, or mayonnaise
10 peanuts

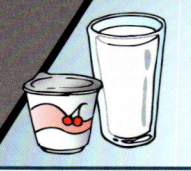

- Eat less fat
- Eat less saturated fat. It is found in meat and animal products such as hamburger, cheese, bacon, and butter

Milk
(2–3 servings)
A serving can be:
1 cup milk
1 cup yogurt

- Choose low-fat or nonfat milk or yogurt
- Yogurt has natural sugar in it. It can also have added sugar or artificial sweeteners. Yogurt with artificial sweetners has fewer calories than yogurt with added sugar

Vegetables
(3–5 servings)
A serving can be:
1 cup raw vegetables
1/2 cup cooked vegetables
1/2 cup tomato or vegetable juice

- Choose fresh or frozen vegetables without added sauces, fats, or salts
- Choose more dark green and dark yellow vegetables, such as spinach, broccoli, romaine, carrots, and peppers

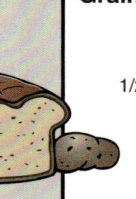

Grains, Beans, & Starchy Vegetables
(6 or more servings)
A serving can be:
1 slice of bread
1/2 small bagel, English muffin, or pita bread
1/2 hamburger or hot dog bun
1 6-inch tortilla
4 to 6 crackers
1/2 cup cooked cereal, pasta, or bulgur
1/3 cup cooked rice
3/4 cup dry cereal
1/2 cup cooked beans, lentils, peas, or corn
1 small potato
1 cup winter squash
1/2 cup sweet potato or yam

How Is Diabetes Treated?

Alcohol:
- If you choose to drink alcohol, limit the amount and have it with a meal. Check with your health professional about a safe amount for you

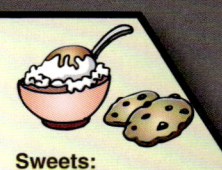

Sweets:
A serving of sweets can be: 1/2 cup ice cream
1 small cupcake or muffin
2 small cookies

- Choose sweets less often because they are high in fat and sugar
- When you do eat sweets, make them part of your healthy diet. Don't eat them as extras

Meat & Others
(2–3 servings)
A serving can be:
2 to 3 oz. of cooked lean meat, poultry, or fish
1/2 to 3/4 cup tuna or cottage cheese
2 to 3 oz. cheese
1 egg*
2 Tbsp. peanut butter
4 oz. tofu*

*equivalent to 1 oz. of meat

- Choose fish and poultry more often. Remove the skin from chicken and turkey
- Select lean cuts of beef, veal, pork, or wild game
- Trim all visible fat from meat
- Bake, roast, broil, grill, or boil instead of frying or adding fat

Fruits
(2–4 servings)
A serving can be:
1 small fresh fruit
1/2 cup canned fruit
1/4 cup dried fruit
1/2 cup fruit juice

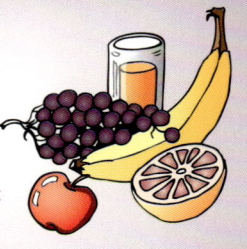

- Choose whole fruits more often than juices. They have more fiber
- Choose fruits and fruit juice without added sweetners or syrups
- Choose citrus fruit such as oranges, grapefruit, or tangerines

- Choose whole-grain foods such as whole-grain bread or crackers, tortillas, bran cereal, brown rice, or bulgur. They're nutritious and high in fiber
- Choose beans as a good source of fiber
- Use whole-wheat or other whole-grain flours in cooking and baking
- Eat more low-fat breads such as bagels, tortillas, English muffins, and pita bread

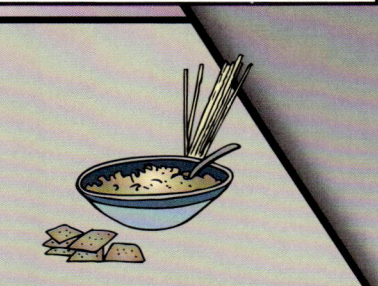

Source: Madigan Army Medical Center, Nutrition Care Division, "The Diabetic Food Pyramid."
www.mamc.amedd.army.mil.

Diabetes

Use of Insulin Versus Oral Medications to Manage Diabetes

People with type 1 diabetes must take multiple injections of insulin on a daily basis to maintain their blood sugar levels in the normal range. People with type 2 diabetes can often control their blood sugar levels using oral medication, diet, exercise, and maintaining normal body weight. However, many people with type 2 diabetes come to need insulin to maintain near normal blood sugar levels. This pie graph shows that most people use oral medication, not insulin, to control their blood sugar levels, which makes sense because over 90 percent of the people with diabetes in the United States, have type 2 diabetes.

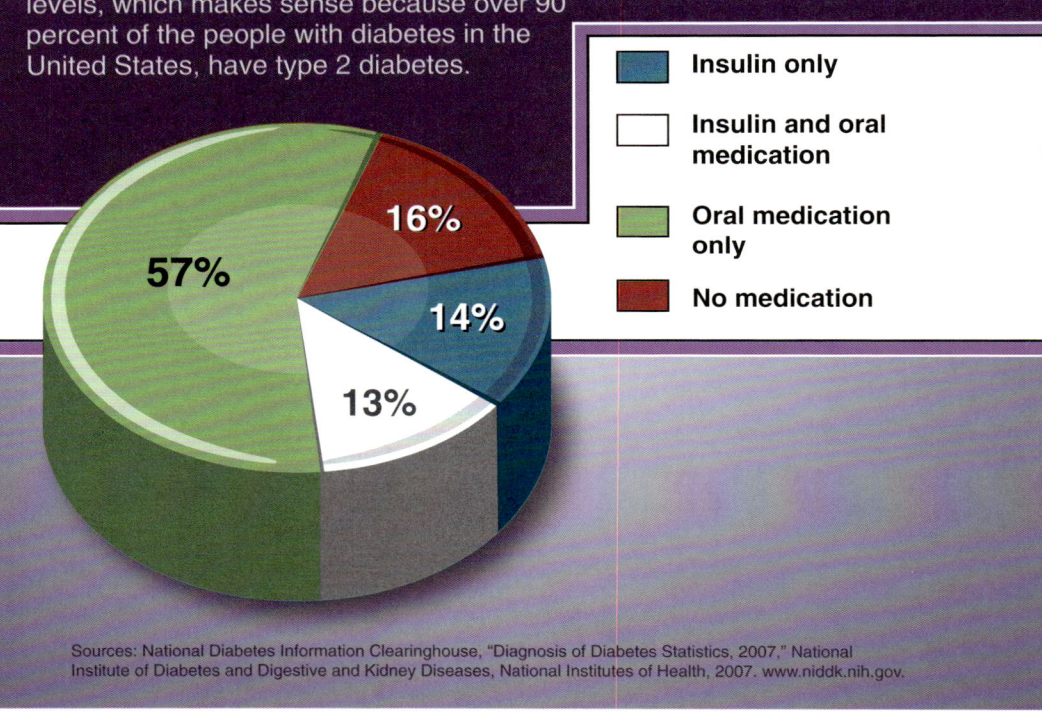

- Insulin only
- Insulin and oral medication
- Oral medication only
- No medication

57%
16%
14%
13%

Sources: National Diabetes Information Clearinghouse, "Diagnosis of Diabetes Statistics, 2007," National Institute of Diabetes and Digestive and Kidney Diseases, National Institutes of Health, 2007. www.niddk.nih.gov.

- **Hypoglycemia** (low blood sugar) is a significant obstacle to obtaining very tight control over blood sugar levels.

- Trial studies show use of a continuous **blood glucose monitor** can help lower blood sugar levels without increasing the risk of hypoglycemia.

How Is Diabetes Treated?

Hypoglycemia and Hyperglycemia

Maintaining a normal blood sugar level is not easy. Blood sugar increases after eating, decreases when exercising, and fluctuates when a person is sick. If a person's blood sugar level drops below 70mg/dl because he or she took too much insulin, missed a meal or snack, or exercised too long or hard, that person can suffer from hypoglycemia or low blood sugar. On the other hand, if blood sugar levels get too high because a person forgot to take medicine, ate too much, got sick, or did not exercise, he or she can suffer from hyperglycemia, or high blood sugar. Not only will hyperglycemia lead to long-term complications of diabetes, but both hypoglycemia and hyperglycemia can be life threatening if not treated.

	Hypoglycemia	*Hyperglycemia*
Common name	Low Blood Sugar	High Blood Sugar
Cause	Blood sugar level below 70 mg/ml	Blood sugar level above 130 mg/ml
Symptoms	Hunger, shakiness, sweating, nervousness, dizziness, confusion, sleepiness, difficulty speaking, anxiety, weakness	Frequent urination, excessive thirst, lack of energy, weight loss, blurred vision. May not have symptoms if the body is used to a high blood sugar level
Onset	Can happen suddenly	Gradual
Treatment	Eat something high in sugar, glucose tablets, 1/2 cup fruit juice or regular soda, 1 cup milk, 5–6 pieces of hard candy, 1 tsp sugar or honey	Eat less, exercise more, adjust insulin or oral medication to better manage blood sugar levels
Danger	Very low blood sugar can cause coma, seizures, even death and is more common in people with type 1 diabetes	Blood sugar levels above 360 mg/dl can lead to coma and death
Who is at risk?	People with diabetes who are taking insulin or oral medication to lower their blood sugar levels. Hypoglycemia is especially dangerous for those with "hypoglycemia unawareness" who do not have the warning symptoms of hypoglycemia and don't know to eat something to raise their blood sugar levels.	People with diabetes whose blood sugar levels are not controlled.

Sources: American Medical Association, ed. Boyd E. Metzger, *Guide to Living with Diabetes*. Hoboken, NJ: Wiley and Sons, 2006; Maria Collazo-Clavell, *Mayo Clinic on Managing Diabetes*. Rochester, MN: Mayo Foundation for Medical Education and Research, 2006; National Diabetes Information Clearinghouse, "Hypoglycemia," National Institute of Diabetes and Digestive and Kidney Diseases, National Institutes of Health. www.niddk.nih.gov; Rosemary Walker and Jill Rodgers in association with the American Diabetes Association, *Diabetes: A Practical Guide to Managing your Health*. New York: Dorling Kindersley, 2004.

Can Diabetes Be Cured?

❝We wish for a cure, yes, because it's a difficult road. Because it's impossibly sad to draw blood eight times a day from a seven-month old infant. Because it's enormously frustrating to do all you can, only to have technology fail you. . . . Because to imagine your beautiful thirteen-year-old with a shortened life span, amputations, or blindness weighs endlessly on a mother's heart.❞

—Gail O'Keefe, mother of two children with diabetes.

❝The ultimate goal is to walk away from devices and cure diabetes.❞

—Aaron J. Kowalski, strategic director of research, Juvenile Diabetes Research Foundation International.

At present, there is no known cure for diabetes. The discovery of insulin in 1922 and advances in science and technology in the following decades have enabled people with diabetes to manage their disease and live active and productive lives. However, a cure for diabetes remains out of reach—for now. Scientists continue to work toward a cure, but in the meantime preventing people from getting the disease is the only way to halt the epidemic of diabetes in America.

Preventing Type 2 Diabetes

Numerous studies have shown that losing weight and engaging in moderate exercise can prevent or delay the onset of type 2 diabetes. The most famous study, the Diabetes Prevention Program (DPP), found that lifestyle changes worked among all ethnic groups and were particularly effective for participants aged 60 years and older. Further analysis found that weight loss was the main factor that reduced the risk for developing diabetes. As Allen Spiegel, director of the National Institute of Diabetes and Digestive and Kidney Diseases, noted, "The DPP findings represent a major step toward the goal of containing and ultimately reversing the epidemic of type 2 diabetes in this country."[30]

A second study, the Malmo Feasibility Study, found that weight loss and exercise helped not only those who had prediabetes, but also those with type 2 diabetes—nearly 50 percent who did not yet have symptoms regained the ability to control their blood sugars. Weight loss and improved fitness each helped increase glucose tolerance, but together, they were even more effective.

Preventing Type 1 Diabetes

Preventing type 1 diabetes remains a challenge. Scientists know type 1 diabetes is an autoimmune disease—that something causes the body's immune system to malfunction and attack and destroy the beta cells of a person's pancreas. But without knowing what triggers the onset of the disease, scientists are stuck searching for ways either to prevent the autoimmune reaction from occurring or to stop the autoimmune reaction once it has begun.

One approach is to strengthen the immune system itself. Building on studies that show common stomach bacteria can protect mice from type 1 diabetes, Li Wen, a research scientist at Yale School of Medicine, notes: "Understanding how gut bacteria work on the immune system to influence whether diabetes and other autoimmune diseases occur is very important. This understanding

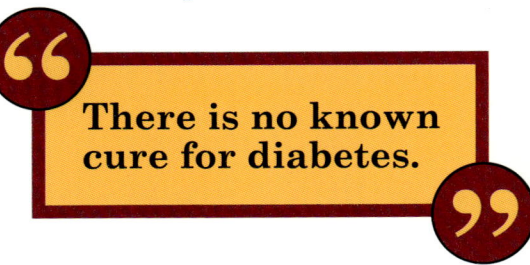

> **There is no known cure for diabetes.**

may allow us to design ways to target the immune system through altering the balance of friendly gut bacteria and protect against diabetes."[31]

Another approach is being taken by a group of Finnish scientists who uncovered changes in fat and protein metabolism among children who later developed type 1 diabetes. If the autoimmune response is a reaction to an underlying metabolic problem, identifying the metabolic problem at an early age and treating it might prevent the onset of type 1 diabetes.

Currently, the presence of antibodies to the beta cells is the first detectable sign that the autoimmune reaction of type 1 diabetes is under way. Treating patients immediately with anti-CD3 antibody, an antibody designed to stop the autoimmune reaction, has had some success. One year after treatment, patients produced more insulin and needed less injected insulin than patients not receiving anti-CD3 antibody. Jeffrey Bluestone at the University of San Francisco thinks that "the antibody may selectively inhibit previously activated immune cells that are involved in the development of diabetes."[32]

Pancreatic and Kidney Transplants

The only way to cure diabetes is to regenerate the body's ability to produce and regulate insulin. Transplanting a healthy pancreas into a person with diabetes is one way to reestablish production of insulin. However, with less than 2,000 donor pancreases available each year, the supply is extremely limited. Pancreatic transplants are usually performed on people who also need a kidney transplant or those with type 1 diabetes who are otherwise healthy but their diabetes cannot be controlled with insulin. To date, the most successful outcomes have occurred in patients receiving a simultaneous pancreatic-kidney transplant. Typically 80 to 85 percent of patients receiving a pancreatic transplant regain the ability to produce and regulate insulin and no longer need injections of insulin.

> **The only way to cure diabetes is to regenerate the body's ability to produce and regulate insulin.**

But organ transplant carries a risk that the new organ will be rejected by the body. People who receive a pancreatic-kidney transplant must use antirejection drugs for life to suppress the body's natural immune response. These drugs often have more negative side effects than continual injections of insulin. Christopher D. Saudek, former president of the American Diabetes Association, warns, "[Pancreatic transplant] surgery is so major and the need for continuous immune suppression is more dangerous than taking insulin."[33] Thus, if insulin is working, there is little justification for taking the risks associated with a pancreatic transplant.

An Artificial Pancreas

An artificial pancreas would monitor a person's blood sugar, calculate when and how much insulin is needed, and deliver the correct dose of insulin, just like a functioning pancreas does. While not a cure for diabetes, an artificial pancreas could improve control of blood sugar levels and provide relief from the constant need to juggle food, insulin, and exercise. Plus, because the system is artificial, it can be designed to avoid the body's natural immune system, thus eliminating the need for antirejection medication.

Two of the components needed to develop an artificial pancreas are currently available: continuous glucose monitors, which continually monitor and record or report blood sugar levels and insulin pumps that deliver insulin via a tube inserted beneath the skin. What is missing is the "brain"—something that can take data from the continuous glucose monitor, use it to predict the amount of insulin that will be needed, and cause the insulin pump to deliver that dose of insulin. Computer models to predict insulin needs are being tested at the City of Hope Hospital in Los Angeles and in Cambridge, England. If scientists can get the computer models to work, an artificial pancreas could be developed within the next five years.

Transplanting Islet Cells

Islet cell transplantation is a less invasive alternative to pancreatic transplants. Instead of transplanting the entire pancreas, the islets containing the beta cells are isolated and removed from one or 2 donor pancreases. The islets are inserted via a small plastic tube, or catheter, next to the large portal vein of the liver, where they have access to a blood supply. Once implanted, the beta cells make and produce insulin, allowing the patient to stop taking insulin injections. Gary Kleiman, 1 of the first 100 patients to receive an islet transplant and a survivor of 2 kidney transplants, found he no longer needed to take 4 to 5 insulin injections each day. Of his surgery, Kleiman says, "It's given my life a tremendous amount of freedom, flexibility, lack of worry and, in truth, it's given me a feeling of having a future."[34]

Islet transplant is haunted by many of the same problems as pancreatic transplants, including the need to take antirejection drugs that suppress the immune system and the limited number of donor pancreases available. In addition, there is the worry that the same autoimmune response that destroyed the original beta cells will also destroy the islets. About 85 percent of patients who receive islet transplantation are free of their insulin injections one year later, but after 2 years only about 33 percent remain insulin independent, dropping to as few as 11 percent 5 years later. Many patients are still able to reduce their need for insulin, achieve better blood sugar control, and reduce problems with hypoglycemia, despite the drop in insulin production by the islets.

Keeping the Islets Alive

Researchers continue to explore why transplanted islets lose their ability to produce insulin and what might ensure that more transplanted islets survive. Most of this work is still in the experimental stage, with scientists exploring a variety of approaches, including how to prevent damage to the islets during transplantation, how to prevent rejection of the transplanted islets, and how to block the underlying autoimmune response that killed the beta cells of the patient's own islets in the first place.

In Sweden researchers have evidence that a buildup of protein, called amyloid, may destroy the transplanted islets. "We previously knew that amyloid production is a symptom of stress that leads to cell death in type 2 diabetes. Perhaps the same thing happens in a transplant, when cells are exposed to great stress,"[35] says Gunilla T. Westermark, lead author of the study. If so, reducing stress on the transplanted cells may help the islets survive longer after implant.

> **If insulin is working, there is little justification for taking the risks associated with a pancreatic transplant.**

In the United States scientists have developed a procedure that could eliminate the need for antirejection drugs when transplanting islet cells. Injecting diabetic mice with treated splenocytes (blood cells from the spleen) from the same donor as the islet cells seven days before the islet cells are transplanted resulted in 70 percent of the islet cells surviving over time. The treated splenocytes seem to prime the immune system to accept the donor islet cells as the body's own. If this technique could be developed to work in humans, it might enable more transplanted islets to survive and eliminate the need for transplant patients to take antirejection medications for life.

A Lack of Donors

Like pancreatic transplants, transplanting islet cells is limited by the number of people who donate their pancreases after they die. "There are simply not enough deceased donors available to meet the demand for islet cells," says Kwang-Won Kim. "In fact, we sometimes require islet cells from two deceased donors to gather enough cells to treat one patient."[36] Living donors would be able to provide many more healthy cells because islet cells deteriorate quickly after death. In samples taken from living donors, 94 percent of the islet cells are viable for transplant, compared with 42 percent of the cells taken from deceased donors. However, obtaining islet cells from living donors may put the donor at risk for developing diabetes.

> **Researchers continue to explore why the transplanted islets lose their ability to produce insulin and what might ensure that more transplanted islets survive.**

Researchers around the world are trying to develop a source of islet cells that could meet the demand for islet transplant. Scientists at the University of Pittsburgh School of Medicine have stimulated human beta cells to reproduce in both the laboratory and in a living animal. "After we transplanted some of these engineered human beta cells under the outer layer of a kidney in a diabetic mouse, we saw that replication continued and blood sugar levels normalized,"[37] said Nathalie Fiaschi-Taesch, a lead author of the study.

Shimon Efrat, a professor at Tel Aviv University's Sackler Faculty of Medicine, has also developed a way to grow human beta cells in the laboratory. "We are able to grow a massive reserve of healthy cells that may be made to produce enough insulin to restore the function of the destroyed cells," says Efrat. "In theory, cells from one donor can be multiplied thousands of times."[38] There still remains the problem of getting the body's immune system to accept the transplanted cells, but these new developments may end the current shortage of islet cells available for transplant.

Regenerating Beta Cells

Denise Faustman at Massachusetts General Hospital and Harvard Medical School concluded that diabetes could not be cured through pancreatic or islet transplants, beta cell replication, or stem cells because none of these methods addressed the underlying problem—the body's autoimmune response to the beta cells. "Diabetes therapy, in the future, could involve the regeneration of insulin-secreting cells . . . [but] neither approach to replenishing islet cells can be curative unless the underlying autoimmune defect is eliminated."[39] Accordingly, she refocused her efforts on the immune system. Using a technique to block the underlying autoimmune response to the beta cells, Faustman transplanted both stem cells from a donor spleen and islets into diabetic mice at the end stage of the disease. Not only did the islet cells survive, but when the islet cells were removed, the mice continued to produce and regulate insulin. Further investigation showed the mice had developed working beta cells within the pancreas. The mice had been cured of diabetes.

Since Faustman published her work in 2001, other researchers have reproduced her results. In 2006 Louis Phillipson, the senior author of a study conducted by the University of Chicago, wrote, "Our studies confirm that autoimmune diabetes can be reversed [in mice with type 1 diabetes]."[40] The same effect has not been proven in humans, but the research suggests that even a long time after mice are diabetic, they have the ability to produce new beta cells. If humans also have the capacity to regenerate beta cells, it could be possible to cure diabetes. The very idea of a potential cure has people with diabetes, their families, and doctors looking toward the future with hope.

Primary Source Quotes*

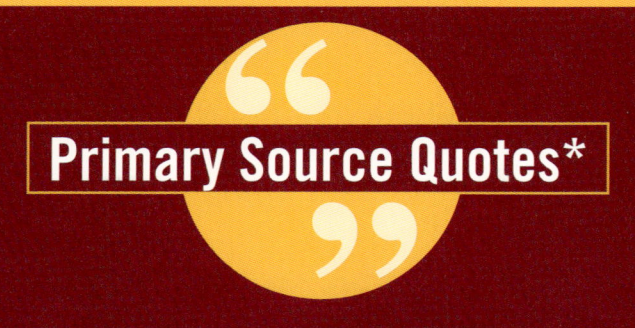

Can Diabetes Be Cured?

> **People in the diabetes community, desperate for a cure, sometimes express considerable paranoia about the goals of the pharmaceutical industry. After all, with $174 billion expended each year for diabetes care in the United States alone, the manufacturers of drugs and diabetes products make serious money off the disease. Do they, then, have any incentive to find a cure for it?**

—Dara Mayers, "Would You Cure a Profitable Disease?" *Diabetes Health*, June 11, 2008.

Mayers is a health-care strategist, writer, and editor.

> **Although that cure [for diabetes] is still elusive, the foundation of information and research continues to grow annually, pushing us toward a cure.**

—American Diabetes Association, "American Diabetes Association Reflects on 2008 Accomplishments in the Fight Against Diabetes and Looks Ahead to Challenges in 2009," press release, Alexandria, VA, January 8, 2009.

The American Diabetes Association funds and advocates for research, publishes scientific findings, advocates for the rights of people with diabetes, and provides information and services to people with diabetes, their families, health-care professionals, and the public.

---

* Editor's Note: While the definition of a primary source can be narrowly or broadly defined, for the purposes of Compact Research, a primary source consists of: 1) results of original research presented by an organization or researcher; 2) eyewitness accounts of events, personal experience, or work experience; 3) first-person editorials offering pundits' opinions; 4) government officials presenting political plans and/or policies; 5) representatives of organizations presenting testimony or policy.

Diabetes

> "Diabetes can now be tamed but it cannot be cured. Someday, I know a cure will be found. . . . I dream of safely curing my insulin-requiring patients, of helping them to live without needles and lancets and the ups and downs of insulin use."

—Anne L. Peters, *Conquering Diabetes: A Cutting-Edge, Comprehensive Program for Prevention and Health*. New York: Hudson Street, 2005.

Peters is a professor of medicine and the director of the University of Southern California's clinical diabetes programs. She is the former chairperson of the American Diabetes Association Council on Health Care Delivery and Public Health.

> "Every disease, in the search for a cure, generates a sine wave of great expectation followed by disillusionment; but in diabetes, the hopes have been higher, the promises more explicit, the disappointment more bitter."

—James S. Hirsch, *Cheating Destiny: Living with Diabetes*. Boston: Houghton Mifflin, 2006.

Hirsch is a former reporter for the *New York Times* and the *Wall Street Journal* who was diagnosed with type 1 diabetes at age 15 and has a son and brother who also have type 1 diabetes.

> "We are actually lucky that we have diabetes rather than some rare disease. Worldwide, about 194 million people have diabetes according to the International Diabetes Federation. That makes diabetes a terribly tempting target for anyone interested in fame, fortune or the opportunity to help mankind."

—David Mendosa, "Curing Diabetes," MyDiabetesCentral.com. www.diabetescentral.com, March 3, 2006.

Mendosa is a medical writer and consultant specializing in diabetes.

Can Diabetes Be Cured?

> "The need for a closed loop system—a fully automated monitor and pump technology [an artificial pancreas]—has never been greater. But it's also never been more technically feasible."

—Aaron J. Kowalski, "Accelerating the Availability of an Artificial Pancreas." Remarks presented at the Eighth Annual Diabetes Technology Meeting in New York, November, 14, 2008.

Kowalski is the strategic director for research at the Juvenile Diabetes Research Foundation International.

> "There's no cure for [diabetes], but you can definitely get it under control."

—"Randy Jackson's Struggle with Diabetes," CBS News, October 1, 2007. www.cbsnews.com.

Jackson is a Grammy-winning musician and a judge on *American Idol*. He has type 2 diabetes and is the spokesperson for the American Heart Association's The Heart of Diabetes Campaign.

> "We've proven that if people eat right, lose weight, and become physically active, they can halt the progression to full-blown diabetes. But . . . health insurance pays for doctor visits, medications, surgeries and hospitalizations. Prevention . . . is another story. Less than 1 percent of the billions spent annually on health care in the United States is spent on prevention."

—Francine Ratner Kaufman, *Diabesity*. New York: Bantam, 2006.

Kaufman is the director of the Comprehensive Childhood Diabetes Center and head of the Center for Endocrinology, Diabetes, and Metabolism at Children's Hospital in Los Angeles.

> "It is crucial to continue basic and clinical research to identify new ways to improve the quality of life of type 1 diabetes patients. . . . Research is the key."

—Allen M. Spiegel, "Recent Developments in Research on Type 1 Diabetes, testimony before the Committee on Homeland Security and Governmental Affairs, U.S. Senate, June 21, 2005.

Spiegel is the director of the National Institute of Diabetes and Digestive and Kidney Diseases, which is part of the National Institutes of Health and funds research on diabetes.

Facts and Illustrations

Can Diabetes Be Cured?

- Less than **1 percent** of the billions spent on health care in this country is spent on prevention.

- **Insulin** is not a cure for diabetes, nor does it prevent the complications of diabetes.

- Success treating **diabetes in mice** does not directly transfer to treatments that work in humans.

- A real cure could emerge from **cell-based therapy**, such as the transplantation of insulin-producing cells, but the underlying autoimmune process must be addressed.

- The lifelong need for drugs to prevent rejection of a transplant is a **barrier** to both pancreatic and islet cell transplants.

- More people survive **pancreatic-kidney transplant** operations with better outcomes than patients who receive only a pancreas transplant.

- About **85 percent** of people who receive a simultaneous pancreas-kidney transplant have a functioning pancreas after one year. The rate drops to about **70 percent** after five years.

- A major barrier that limits the widespread use of islet transplantation is an **inadequate supply of islets**.

Can Diabetes Be Cured?

Federal Spending on Disease Research (in Millions)

Research/Disease Areas	2008
Cancer	$5,570
HIV/AIDS	$2,928
Cardiovascular	$2,027
Vaccine Related	$1,632
Obesity	$664
Alzheimer's Disease	$412
Diabetes	**$402**
Depression	$402
Hepatitis	$180
Multiple Sclerosis	$169
Epilepsy	$145
Autism	$118
Attention Deficit Disorder (ADD)	$60
HPV and/or Cervical Cancer Vaccines	$19
Down Syndrome	$17
Anorexia	$7

Source: NIH Research Portfolio Online Reporting Tool (RePORT). http://report.nih.gov.

Diabetes

Pancreatic Islet Transplantation

Harvesting islets from a donor pancreas and transplanting the islets rather than the entire pancreas is a much easier operation. The entire procedure takes less than an hour. Patients remain awake while the islets are inserted via a small plastic tube or catheter to a spot next to the large vein of the liver. Full islet function and new blood vessel growth take time, but for most patients, the insulin produced by the transplanted islets do the job of the beta cells that were destroyed by the autoimmune reaction of type 1 diabetes. This allows the patient to stop taking insulin. Unfortunately, the transplanted islet cells die off over time, leaving the patient dependant again of insulin injections for survival. Scientists are working to find a way to keep the islets alive.

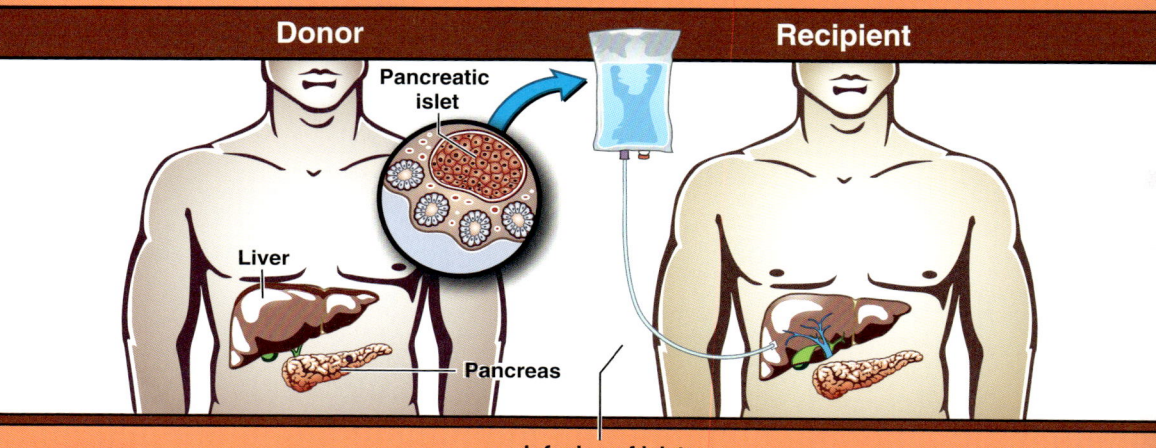

Donor — Pancreatic islet — Liver — Pancreas

Recipient

Infusion of islets

Sources: National Diabetes Information Clearinghouse, "Pancreatic Islet Transplantation," National Diabetes Statistics, 2007, National Institute of Diabetes & Digestive & Kidney Diseases, National Institutes of Health. http://diabetes.niddk.nih.gov.

- Less than **2,000** donor pancreases are available for transplant each year.

- It takes up to **two donor pancreases** to gather enough islets for an islet cell transplant.

- About **85 percent** of patients who receive islet transplantation are insulin free 1 year later. The rate drops to around **11 percent** after 5 years.

Can Diabetes Be Cured?

Obesity Operation Cures Diabetes in Some Patients

Australian researchers say that morbidly obese patients who undergo stomach band surgery are 5 times more likely to see the illness disappear over a 2-year period than those who have standard diabetes care. According to the researchers most of the surgery patients were able to stop using diabetes drugs and even acheived normal blood tests. After 2 years the surgery patients lost an average of 46 pounds (20.9kg), which reduced diabetes symptoms or eliminated the illness.

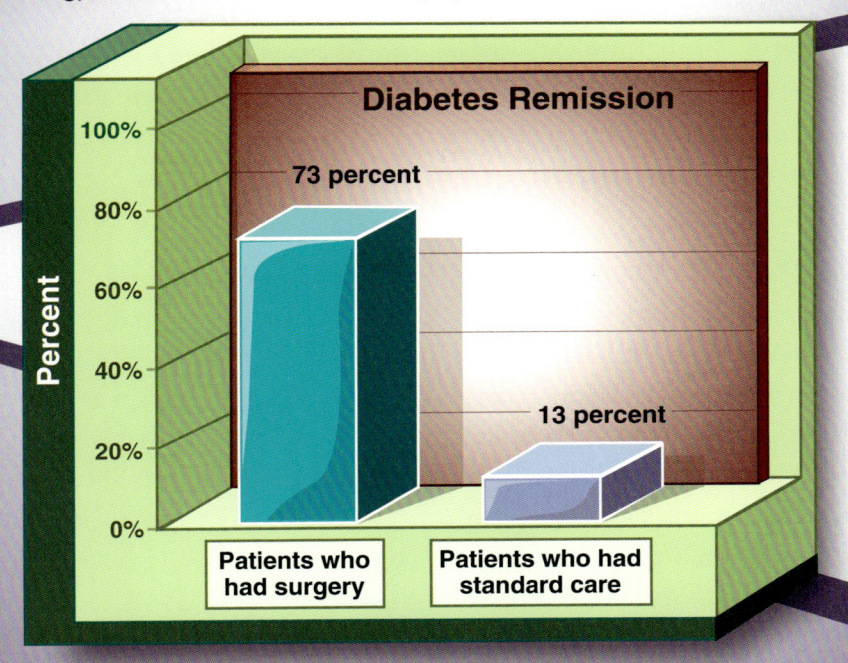

Diabetes Remission

Patients who had surgery	Patients who had standard care
73 percent	13 percent

Source: MSNBC, "Obesity Operation May Cure Diabetes in Many," January 22, 2008. www.msnbc.msn.com.

Key People and Advocacy Groups

American Diabetes Association: Founded to prevent and cure diabetes and improve the lives of all people affected by the disease, the association funds and advocates for research, publishes scientific findings, advocates for the rights of people with diabetes, and provides information and services to people with diabetes, their families, health-care professionals, and the public.

Jeffrey A. Bluestone: Bluestone is the director of the Diabetes Center at the University of California–San Francisco and the Immune Tolerance Network. His research focuses on understanding immune responses to transplants and autoantigens.

Mayer B. Davidson: Davidson is a professor of medicine at the University of California–Los Angeles School of Medicine, a past president of the American Diabetes Association, and the director of the Center for Urban Research and Education in Diabetes and Metabolism at Charles Drew University. In 1998 he started a nurse-directed diabetes program in the low-income area of south central Los Angeles that is able to provide the patient support needed for low-income patients to maintain control of their diabetes. He is also the author of *The Complete Idiot's Guide to Diabetes*.

Steven V. Edelman: Edelman is a professor of medicine at the University of California–San Diego School of Medicine, Veterans Affairs Medical Center, and the founder and director of the national organization Taking Control of Your Diabetes, which assists patients with managing their diabetes. Diagnosed with diabetes at the age of 15, Edelman has become a local and national leader in diabetes treatment, research, and education.

Key People and Advocacy Groups

Denise L. Faustman: Faustman is the director of the Immunobiology Laboratory at Massachusetts General Hospital and an associate professor of medicine at Harvard Medical School. Her research includes modifying antigens on donor tissues to prevent their rejection and working to uncover new treatments for curing type 1 diabetes. She was the subject of much controversy when her lab reversed type 1 diabetes in mice with end-stage disease, but subsequent studies have now replicated her results.

Irl B. Hirsch: Hirsch is a professor of medicine in the Division of Metabolism, Endocrinology, and Nutrition at the University of Washington School of Medicine. Diagnosed with type 1 diabetes at age six, his research focuses on using new technologies to improve diabetes therapy, particularly the use of real-time continuous glucose sensors and how changes in blood sugar levels impact the development of diabetes-related complications.

James S. Hirsch: A former reporter for the *New York Times* and the *Wall Street Journal* and the author of *Cheating Destiny: Living with Diabetes*, Hirsch was diagnosed with type 1 diabetes at age 15 and has a son and brother who also have type 1 diabetes.

Joan Williams Hoover: An advocate for people with diabetes and the mother of a child with diabetes who suffered numerous severe complications before dying at age 15, Hoover was one of the first people to articulate the concept of diabetes burnout.

Juvenile Diabetes Research Foundation International: The foundation was originally created by a group of parents advocating for their children with diabetes and called the Juvenile Diabetes Foundation. Now an international organization, the foundation's mission is to find a cure for diabetes and its complications by funding research in the restoration of normal blood sugar levels, avoidance and reversal of complications, and prevention of diabetes and its recurrence.

Francine Ratner Kaufman: Kaufman is the director of the Comprehensive Childhood Diabetes Center and head of the Center for Endocrinology, Diabetes, and Metabolism at Children's Hospital in Los Angeles and a past president of the American Diabetes Association. She is the current chair for the National Diabetes Education Program sponsored by the National Institutes of Health and the Centers for Disease Control and Prevention.

Gary Kleiman: Executive director for medical development at the University of Miami's Diabetes Research Institute, Kleiman was diagnosed with diabetes at age 6, began going blind at age 18, and has only limited vision now. He had two kidney transplants by the time he was 53 and is doing well with the islet transplant he received November 1, 2002, but is considering having another islet transplant before his current islets die completely.

Florene Linnen: Linnen has type 2 diabetes and has been nicknamed the "Diabetes Queen" for her work to help the mostly African American residents of her community in Georgetown, South Carolina, learn about their disease and demand appropriate health care from their doctors.

David M. Nathan: Nathan is a professor of medicine at Harvard Medical School and the director of the Diabetes Center at Massachusetts General Hospital. He is also an author of the books *Beating Diabetes* and *Every Woman's Guide to Diabetes*.

Anne L. Peters: Peters is a professor of medicine and the director of the University of Southern California's clinical diabetes programs. She is the former chairperson of the American Diabetes Association

Council on Health Care Delivery and Public Health and author of *Conquering Diabetes*.

William H. Polonsky: Polonsky is an assistant clinical professor in psychiatry at the University of California–San Diego and an active researcher in behavioral medicine. He became the first psychologist on the staff of the Joslin Diabetes Center in Boston and is the author of *Diabetes Burnout: What to Do When You Can't Take It Anymore*.

Robert S. Sherwin: Sherwin is the director of the Diabetes Endocrinology Research Center and the Juvenile Diabetes Research Foundation Center for the Study of Hypoglycemia at Yale University and a past president of the Diabetes Association. His special interests include type 1 diabetes, intensified insulin therapy, and hypoglycemia.

Gerald I. Shulman: Shulman is a professor of medicine and cellular and molecular physiology at Yale University. He has received numerous awards for scientific achievement and is a leading authority on insulin resistance, managing type 2 diabetes, and the impact of exercise on the management of diabetes.

Chronology

1500 B.C.
Diabetes is recognized as a disease by the Egyptians.

A.D. 1000
Avicenna, the great Arab physician, records the symptoms and complications of diabetes in his medical encyclopedia, concluding diabetes is incurable.

1901
Eugene Opie of the United States proves the connection between the islets of Langerhans and diabetes.

1938
Long-acting protamine zinc insulin is developed, enabling patients to take one injection of insulin a day.

1952
Lente insulin is introduced; it lasts for up to 30 hours in the body.

1879
Oscar Minowski of Germany unintentionally produces diabetes by removing a dog's pancreas.

1914
Fredrick Allen of the United States introduces his starvation diet, which keeps diabetic patients alive before the discovery of insulin.

1923
Eli Lilly produces huge batches of insulin for human use.

1956
Oral medications, the sulfonylureas, are developed for people with type 2 diabetes.

1922
Frederick Banting, Charles H. Best, J.J.R. Macleod, and James Bertram Collip of Canada announce their discovery of insulin; Nicolas C. Paulesco of Romania published his discovery of insulin two years earlier but got no credit.

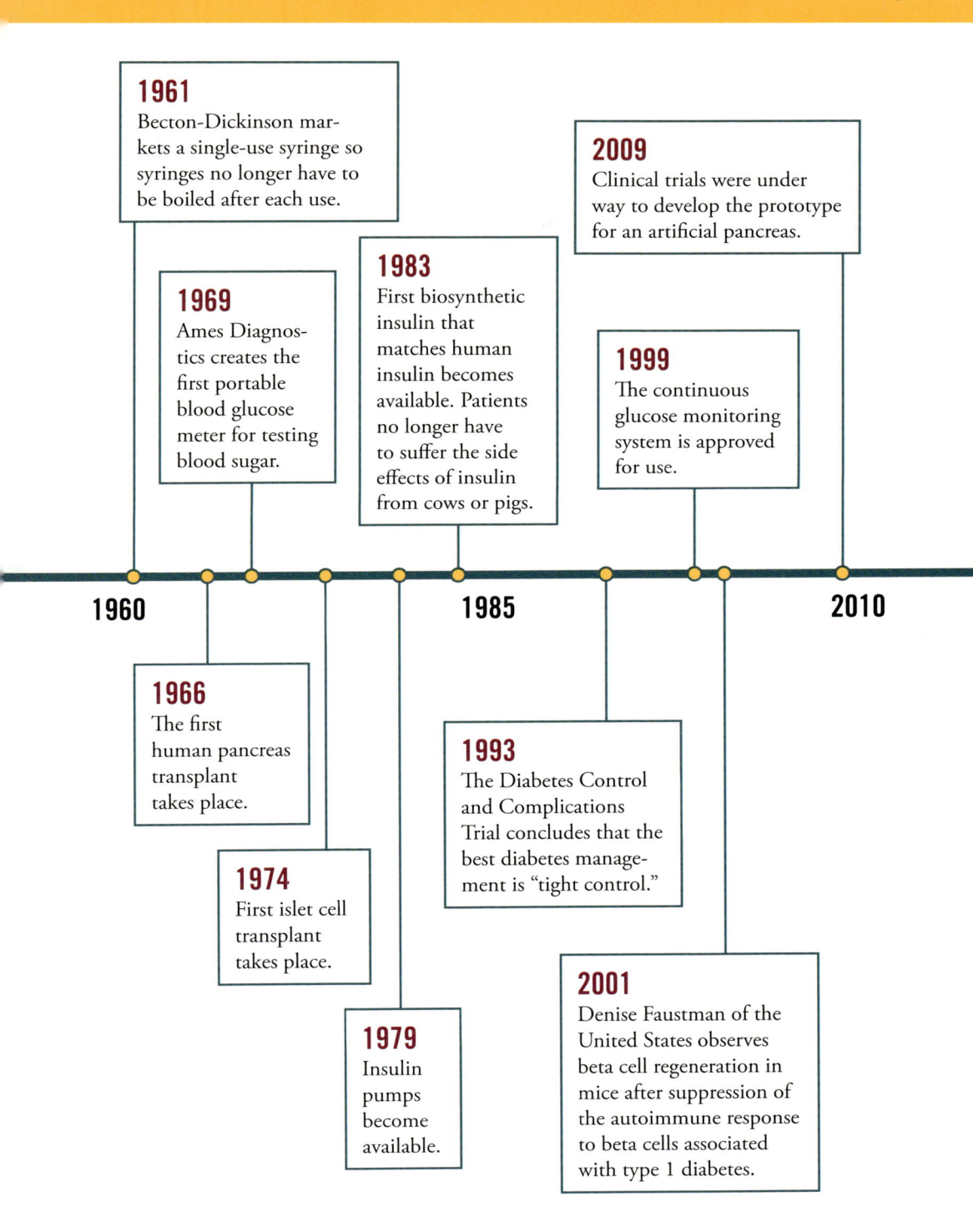

Chronology

1961
Becton-Dickinson markets a single-use syringe so syringes no longer have to be boiled after each use.

1969
Ames Diagnostics creates the first portable blood glucose meter for testing blood sugar.

1983
First biosynthetic insulin that matches human insulin becomes available. Patients no longer have to suffer the side effects of insulin from cows or pigs.

2009
Clinical trials were under way to develop the prototype for an artificial pancreas.

1999
The continuous glucose monitoring system is approved for use.

1960 — 1985 — 2010

1966
The first human pancreas transplant takes place.

1974
First islet cell transplant takes place.

1979
Insulin pumps become available.

1993
The Diabetes Control and Complications Trial concludes that the best diabetes management is "tight control."

2001
Denise Faustman of the United States observes beta cell regeneration in mice after suppression of the autoimmune response to beta cells associated with type 1 diabetes.

Related Organizations

American Diabetes Association

ATTN: National Call Center
1701 N. Beauregard St.
Alexandria, VA 22311
phone: (800) 342-2383
Web site: www.diabetes.org

The American Diabetes Association was founded to prevent and cure diabetes and improve the lives of all people affected by the disease. The association funds and advocates for research, publishes scientific findings, advocates for the rights of people with diabetes, and provides information and services to people with diabetes, their families, health-care professionals, and the public.

Centers for Disease Control and Prevention (CDC)

1600 Clifton Rd.
Atlanta, GA 30333
phone: (800) 232-4636 • TTY: (888) 232-6348
e-mail: cdcinfo@cdc.gov • Web site: www.cdc.gov/diabetes

The CDC is a part of the U.S. Department of Health and Human Services and works to conduct and support public health activities in the United States, including gathering data and funding research, intervention, and health promotion programs. The CDC works to bring together the knowledge and tools people and communities need to protect their health and prevent disease.

Children with Diabetes

8216 Princeton-Glendale Rd., PMB 200
West Chester, OH 45069-1675
Web site: www.childrenwithdiabetes.com

Children with Diabetes operates one of the most-established, well-trafficked online diabetes communities on its Web site, promotes the Quilt for Life diabetes awareness project, and hosts Friends for Life conferences to provide education and support for children with diabetes and their families. Jeff Hitchcock, founder and president, has a daughter who was diagnosed with type 1 diabetes when she was two, and he developed Children with Diabetes to help families dealing with diabetes.

Diabetes Health

PO Box 395
Woodacre, CA 94973-0395
phone: (415) 488-1141 • fax: (415) 488-1922
Web site: www.diabeteshealth.com

Diabetes Health (formerly *Diabetes Interview*) is an online magazine designed to provide the diabetes community with quick and direct access to the latest information from diabetes experts. It tackles the hard questions that plague people with diabetes and is run by people who have firsthand experience with diabetes. In 2004 it was nominated for a Maggie Award by the Western Publications Association.

International Diabetes Federation (IDF)

Avenue Emile De Mot 19
B-1000 Brussels, Belgium
phone: +32-2-5385511 • fax: +32-2-5385114
Web site: www.idf.org

The IDF is a worldwide alliance of over 200 diabetes associations in more than 160 countries. The federation works to bring together people with diabetes and their families, professionals involved in diabetes health care and related fields, diabetes representative organizations, and partners from commercial organizations to raise global awareness of diabetes and promote diabetes care, prevention, and cure. The IDF is associated with the Department of Public Information of the United Nations and has official relations with the World Health Organization and the Pan American Health Organization.

Juvenile Diabetes Research Foundation International

120 Wall St.
New York, NY 10005-4001
phone: (800) 533- 2873
fax: (212) 785-9595
e-mail: info@jdrf.org • Web site: www.jdrf.org

Diabetes

The Juvenile Diabetes Research Foundation was originally created by a group of parents advocating for their children with diabetes and was called the Juvenile Diabetes Foundation. The organization's mission is to find a cure for diabetes and its complications by funding research in the restoration of normal blood sugar levels, avoidance and reversal of complications, and prevention of diabetes and its recurrence.

National Diabetes Education Program

One Diabetes Way
Bethesda, MD 20814-9692
phone: (301) 496-3583
e-mail: ndep@mail.nih.gov • Web site: www.ndep.nih.gov

The National Diabetes Education Program is a federally funded program sponsored by the National Institutes of Health and the Centers for Disease Control and Prevention and includes over 200 partners at the federal, state, and local levels working together to reduce death and disability associated with diabetes. The group focuses on increasing awareness and prevention through lifestyle change, the need to address prediabetes, and the need to improve health care.

National Diabetes Information Clearinghouse

1 Information Way
Bethesda, MD 20892-3560
phone: (800) 860-8747 • TTY: (866) 569-1162 • fax: (703) 738-4929
e-mail: ndic@info.niddk.nih.gov
Web site: www.diabetes.niddk.nih.gov

The National Diabetes Information Clearinghouse collects resource information about diabetes for the National Institute of Diabetes and Digestive and Kidney Disorders (NIDDK) Reference Collection. The clearinghouse provides information about diabetes to people with diabetes and their families, health-care professionals, and the public. The clearinghouse answers questions, develops and distributes publications, and works closely with professionals, patient organizations, and government agencies to coordinate resources about diabetes. Publications produced by the clearinghouse are carefully reviewed by both NIDDK scientists and outside experts.

Related Organizations

National Institute of Diabetes and Digestive and Kidney Disorders (NIDDK)

Building 31, Room 9A06
31 Center Dr., MSC 2560
Bethesda, MD 20892-2560
phone: (301) 496-3583
Web site: www.niddk.nih.gov

The NIDDK is part of the National Institutes of Health and funds basic and clinical research through investigator-initiated grants, program project and center grants, and career development and training awards. The institute also supports research and development projects and large-scale clinical trials.

Taking Control of Your Diabetes (TCOYD)

1110 Camino Del Mar, Suite B
Del Mar, CA 92014
phone: (800) 998-2693 or (858) 755-5683 • fax: (858) 755-6854
Web site: www.tcoyd.org

TCOYD is guided by the belief that every person with diabetes has the right to live a healthy, happy, and productive life. Founded by Steven V. Edelman, a physician who was diagnosed with diabetes at age 15, TCOYD works to educate and motivate people with diabetes to take a more active role in their condition and to provide innovative and integrative continuing diabetes education to medical professionals caring for people with diabetes.

For Further Research

Books
Maria Collazo-Clavell, *Mayo Clinic on Managing Diabetes*. Rochester, MN: Mayo Foundation for Medical Education and Research, 2006.

Laura Hieronymus and Christine Tobin, *Eight Weeks to Maximizing Diabetes Control: How to Improve Your Blood Glucose and Stay Healthy with Type 2 Diabetes*. Alexandria, VA: American Diabetes Association, 2008.

Elaine Magee, *Tell Me What to Eat If I Have Type II Diabetes*. New York: Rosen, 2009.

David G. Marrero, *1000 Years of Diabetes Wisdom*. Alexandria, VA: American Diabetes Association, 2008.

Tom Metcalf, *Perspectives on Diseases and Disorders: Diabetes*. Detroit: Greenhaven, 2007.

Boyd E. Metzger, ed., *American Medical Association Guide to Living with Diabetes*. Hoboken, NJ: Wiley, 2006.

Katrina Parker, *Living with Diabetes*. New York: Checkmark, 2008.

Alan L. Rubin, *Type I Diabetes for Dummies*. Hoboken, NJ: Wiley, 2008.

Virginia Valentine, June Biermann, and Barbara Toohey, *Diabetes: The New Type II*. Jeremy P. Tarcher/Penguin, 2008.

Periodicals
Billy Baker, "A History of Being Innovative and Fun," *Boston Globe*, March 3, 2008.

N.R. Kleinfield, "Diabetes and Its Awful Toll Quietly Emerge as a Crisis," *New York Times*, January 9, 2006.

Daniela Lamas, "Transplant Gives Patient a Future," *Miami Herald*, February 10, 2004.

Dara Mayers, "Would You Cure a Profitable Disease?" *Diabetes Health*, June 11, 2008.

For Further Research

Robert Nohle, "Understanding Diabetes Is Important," *Seattle Post-Intelligencer*, January 5, 2009.

Carol M. Ostrom, "Curing What Ails Us: At the Center of Fixing Our Medical Mess, Primary Care Becomes the Patient," *Seattle Times*, January 18, 2009.

Kyle Peveto, "Study Finds Diabetes More Prevalent in Rural Areas," *Beaumont (TX) Enterprise*, December 19, 2008.

Jeff Roberts, "On Top of Their Game: Three Multi-sort Athletes Up to Challenge of Balancing Diabetes," *Bergen County (NJ) Record*, January 5, 2009.

ScienceDaily, "Coming Epidemic of Type 2 Diabetes in Young Adults," July 12, 2008.

Robert Tanenberg, "Insulin for Type 2 Diabetes: Who, When, and Why?" *Diabetes Health*, November 29, 2007.

Internet Sources

American Diabetes Association, "Alternative Insulin Delivery Systems." www.diabetes.org/for-parents-and-kids/diabetes-care/alternative-insulin.jsp.

Jan Chait, "Trying to Control the Uncontrollable," Diabetes Self-Management, November 7, 2006. www.diabetesselfmanagement.com/blog/Jan_Chait/Trying_to_Control_the_Uncontrollable.

Miranda Hitti, "Treating Type 2 Diabetes ASAP Pays Off," WebMD, September 10, 2008. www.diabetes.webmd.com/news/20080910/treating-type-2-diabetes-asap-pays-off.

National Diabetes Information Clearinghouse, "Diagnosis of Diabetes." www.diabetes.niddk.nih.gov/dm/pubs/diagnosis/index.htm.

National Diabetes Information Clearinghouse, "National Diabetes Statistics, 2007." www.diabetes.niddk.nih.gov/dm/pubs/statistics/index.htm.

Crystal Phend, "ADA: Type 2 Diabetes' Reach into Childhood Defined," MedPage Today, June 26, 2007. www.medpagetoday.com/Endocrinology/Diabetes/6031.

Source Notes

Overview
1. Stanley Mirsky and Joan Rattner Heilman, *Controlling Diabetes the Easy Way*. New York: Random House, 1998, p. 10.
2. Francine Ratner Kaufman, *Diabesity*. New York: Bantam, 2006, p. 43.
3. Quoted in *ScienceDaily*, "Coming Epidemic of Type 2 Diabetes in Young Adults," July 12, 2008. www.sciencedaily.com.
4. Quoted in Carol Lewis, "Diabetes: A Growing Public Health Concern," *FDA Consumer*, January/February 2002. www.fda.gov.
5. Quoted in U.S. Department of Health and Human Services, "HHS Launches New Campaign to Curb Growing Diabetes Epidemic in Hispanics," November 13, 2003. www.hhs.gov.
6. Quoted in National Institute of Diabetes and Digestive and Kidney Diseases, "Studies Yield Key Insights in Preventing Destruction of Insulin-Producing Cells," May 29, 2002, p. 2. www.niddk.nih.gov.

How Serious Is Diabetes?
7. Quoted in Kaufman, *Diabesity*, p. 11.
8. Quoted in Kaufman, *Diabesity*, p. 12.
9. Quoted in James S. Hirsch, *Cheating Destiny: Living with Diabetes*. Boston: Houghton Mifflin, 2006, p. 21.
10. Quoted in Mike Klis, "Broncos Briefs (SPORTS)," *Denver Post*, January 23, 2009.
11. William H. Polonsky, *Diabetes Burnout: What to Do When You Can't Take It Anymore*. Alexandria, VA: American Diabetes Association, 1999, p. viii.
12. N.R. Kleinfield, "Diabetes and Its Awful Toll Quietly Emerge as a Crisis," *New York Times*, January 9, 2006. http://query.nytimes.com.
13. Quoted in ADVANCE, "ADVANCE Trial—Quotable Quotes." www.advance-trial.com.
14. Boyd E. Metzger, ed., *American Medical Association Guide to Living with Diabetes*. Hoboken, NJ: Wiley, 2006, p. 17.
15. Kleinfield, "Diabetes and Its Awful Toll Quietly Emerge as a Crisis."
16. Quoted in University of Michigan Health System, "Press Release: More Young Adults with Diabetes Hospitalized, Costing Billions," November 27, 2007. www.med.umich.edu.

What Causes Diabetes?
17. Quoted in *St Louis (MO) Post-Dispatch*, "Anonymous Family Helps Man on Transplant List," December 25, 2008, p. B9.
18. Maria Collazo-Clavell, *Mayo Clinic on Managing Diabetes*. Rochester, MN: Mayo Foundation for Medical Education and Research, 2006, p. 10.
19. Metzger, *American Medical Association Guide to Living with Diabetes*, p. 21.
20. Quoted in Hirsch, *Cheating Destiny*, p. 16.
21. Kaufman, *Diabesity*, p. 41.

How Is Diabetes Treated?
22. Kaufman, *Diabesity*, pp. 59–60.
23. Richard S. Beaser and Joan V.C. Hill, *The Joslin Guide to Diabetes*. New York: Simon and Schuster, 1995, pp. 109–110.
24. Hirsch, *Cheating Destiny*, p. 122.
25. Metzger, *American Medical Association*

Source Notes

Guide to Living with Diabetes, p. 123.
26. Quoted in Kaufman, *Diabesity*, p. 209.
27. Quoted in Collazo-Clavell, *Mayo Clinic on Managing Diabetes*, p. 39.
28. Quoted in Polonsky, *Diabetes Burnout*, p. 4.
29. Quoted in Hirsch, *Cheating Destiny*, p. 242.

Can Diabetes Be Cured?
30. Quoted in National Institute of Diabetes and Digestive and Kidney Diseases, "Diet and Exercise Dramatically Delay Type 2 Diabetes: Diabetes Medication Metformin Also Effective." www.niddk.nih.gov.
31. Li Wen et al., "Innate Immunity and Intestinal Microbiota in the Development of Type 1 Diabetes," *Nature*, October 23, 2008, pp. 1,109–1,113.
32. Quoted in National Institute of Diabetes and Digestive and Kidney Diseases, "Studies Yield Key Insights in Preventing Destruction of Insulin-Producing Cells," May 29, 2002, p. 2. www.niddk.nih.gov.
33. Quoted in Lewis, "Diabetes."
34. Quoted in NBC Miami, "University of Miami Leading the Way in the Fight Against Diabetes," January 5, 2004. www.nbc6.net.
35. Quoted in *ScienceDaily*, "Why Transplanted Insulin Cells Die," August 28, 2008. www.sciencedaily.com.
36. Quoted in *ScienceDaily*, "Living Donors May Be Best Source of Insulin-Producing Islets for Diabetes Treatment," November 27, 2007. www.sciencedaily.com.
37. Quoted in *ScienceDaily*, "Diabetes: Human Beta Cells Can Be Easily Induced to Replicate," January 15, 2009. www.sciencedaily.com.
38. Quoted in *ScienceDaily*, "Battling Diabetes with Beta Cells," September 3, 2008. www.sciencedaily.com.
39. Shohta Kodama and Denise L. Faustman, "Routes to Regenerating Islet Cells: Stem Cells and Other Biological Therapies for Type 1 Diabetes," *Pediatric Diabetes*, 2004, p. 42.
40. Quoted in Hirsch, *Cheating Destiny*, p. 218.

List of Illustrations

How Serious Is Diabetes?
Number of People with Diabetes Growing	31
Diabetes Has Many Complications	32
The Cost of Diabetes	33

What Causes Diabetes?
Race and Diabetes	45
The Pancreas and Diabetes	46
Characteristics of Type 1 and Type 2 Diabetes	47

How Is Diabetes Treated?
Diabetes Food Pyramid	60–61
Use of Insulin Versus Oral Medications to Manage Diabetes	62
Hypoglycemia and Hyperglycemia	63

Can Diabetes Be Cured?
Federal Spending on Disease Research (in Millions)	75
Pancreatic Islet Transplantation	76
Obesity Operation Cures Diabetes in Some Patients	77

Index

acidosis, 10
adults
   diabetes as leading cause for blindness among, 12
   diabetics, percent meeting blood sugar goals, 59
   growth of diabetes in, 31 (chart)
   type 2 diabetes as percent of all diabetes cases in, 44
   young, type 2 diabetes epidemic among, 26
alpha-glucosidase inhibitors, 50
American Diabetes Association, 29, 60, 71
   on annual cost of diabetes, 22
   on percent of diabetics failing to monitor blood glucose, 53
American Diabetic Association, 60
anti-CD3 antibody, 18–19, 66
autoimmune reaction, in type 1 diabetes, 13
   detection of, 66

Beaser, Richard S., 42, 51
beta cells
   growth of, in laboratory, 69–70
   regeneration of, 70
   in type 1 vs. type 2 diabetes, 41
biguanides, 50
blindness, 24
   blood glucose control in lowering risk of, 49
   diabetes as leading cause for among adults, 12
   number of annual new cases due to diabetes, 33
blood glucose
   control of, 52
   exercise helps stabilize, 52
   importance of controlling, 14–15
   monitoring, 59
   normal levels of, 48
   regulation of, 34–35
blood glucose monitors, 16–17
   continuous, 62
blood vessels, effects of diabetes on, 24
Bluestone, Jeffrey, 66

Campbell, Amy P., 42
cell-based therapy, 74
Centers for Disease Control and Prevention (CDC), 11
Chait, Jan, 58
Chalmers, John, 24
children
   diagnosis of type 2 diabetes in, 41
   number diagnosed with diabetes annually, 30
Clute, Heather Nielsen, 42
Cutler, Jay, 22–23

Delahanty, Linda M., 27, 43, 57
diabetes
   causes of, 13
   complications of, 12, 23–24, 28, 32 (illustration)
      blood glucose control decreases risks of, 52
   cure for, pharmaceutical companies lack incentives to find, 71
   definition of, 8–9
   diagnosis of, 48
   famous people with, 54
   growth in number of adults with, 31 (chart)
   management of, 22–23
   percent of affected adults meeting blood sugar goals, 59
   prevalence of, 6, 11, 30
   race/ethnicity and, 44, 45 (chart)
   risk factors for, 12
   societal burden of, 29
   treatment of, 14–15
   type 1 vs. type 2, 6, 10
      characteristics of, 47 (chart)
      prevalence of, 21–22
   undiagnosed, number of people with, 21
   See also type 1 diabetes; type 2 diabetes
diabetes burnout, 53–54
Diabetes Control and Complications Trial, 14, 49, 59
Diabetes Prevention Program (DPP), 39, 45, 64–65
diabetic coma, 16
diagnosis, 48
diet(s)
   in control of type 2 diabetes, 10
   depend on type of diabetes, 51–52
   difficulty in maintaining, 53

93

Diabetes

food pyramid, 60–61 (illustration)
Dowden, Irma, 34

Edelman, Steven V., 56
Efrat, Shimon, 69–70
Eichten, Chuck, 20
Eisenstat, Stephanie A., 42
exercise, 7
   difficulty in maintaining, 53
   effects on blood sugar levels, 48–49, 52

fat, visceral, metabolic syndrome and, 39–40
Faustman, Denise, 70
Fiaschi-Taesch, Nathalie, 69
food pyramid, for diabetics, 60–61 (illustration)

Galson, Steven, 29
gestational diabetes, 38
   risk for women of developing diabetes after, 46
glucose, 34
   See also blood glucose
glycemic index, 51
glycogen, 8, 15, 34

Hall, Gary, Jr., 53–54
heredity
   link between environment and, research on, 40
   in type 2 diabetes, 13
Herold, Kevan, 19
Hill, Joan V.C., 51
Hirsch, James S., 20, 27
   on diabetes as demonstrating divide between have vs. have-nots in medical care, 58
   on diet and insulin, 51
   on hopes/disappointments generated by search for diabetes cure, 72
   on self-discipline required by diabetics, 48
   on type 1 vs. type 2 diabetes, 41
Holston, Wess, 36
hyperglycemia, comparison with hypoglycemia, 63 (table)
hypoglycemia, 50–51, 62
   comparison with hyperglycemia, 63 (table)
   as obstacle to blood sugar control, 62

insulin, 8
   in control of diabetes, 16
   improvements in delivery of, 17
   methods of taking, 49–50
   types of, 49
   use of, vs. oral medications, 62 (chart)
insulin deficiency, 44
insulin resistance, 44
   type 2 diabetes beginning as, 43
insulin-dependent diabetes. *See* type 1 diabetes
insulin-resistance syndrome. *See* metabolic syndrome
International Diabetes Federation, 72
islet transplantation, 17–18, 67, 76 (illustration)
   limited number of donors for, 69–70, 74
   success rate of, 68, 74, 76
islets of Langerhans, 9
   research on, 68–69

The Joslin Guide to Diabetes (Hill), 51
juvenile diabetes. *See* type 1 diabetes

Kaufman, Francine Ratner, 43, 49
   on burden of diabetics, 55
   on complications of untreated diabetes, 12
   on lack of resources for prevention, 73
   on metabolic syndrome, 39
   on need for health-care reform, 29
ketoacidosis, 51, 56
kidney failure, percent caused by diabetes, 12, 33
kidney-pancreatic transplants, 17, 66–67
   success of, 74
Kim, Kwang-Won, 69
Kleiman, Gary, 67
Kleinfield, N.R., 23, 25–26
Kowalski, Aaron J., 64, 73

Langerhans, Paul, 9
Lee, Joyce, 14, 26
Levbarg, Adam M., 55
life expectancy, of people with diabetes vs. general population, 31

Malmo Feasibility Study, 65
Marple, Katherine, 56
Mayers, Dara, 71
medical costs, 30
   avoidable, from variations in care, 59
   of diabetes, 22
      annually, 30
      by type of care, 33 (chart)
   percent spent on disease prevention, 74

Index

meglitinides, 50
Mendosa, David, 72
metabolic syndrome, 6–7, 39–40
Metzger, Boyd E., 25, 52, 57
Mirsky, Stanley, 10

Nathan, David M., 27, 43, 57
National Center for Chronic Disease Prevention and Health Promotion, 41
National Committee for Quality Assurance, 59
National Diabetes Information Clearinghouse, 21
National Institute of Diabetes and Digestive and Kidney Diseases, 28, 43
National Institutes of Health (NIH), 18
Nauruans (Pacific island peoples), 25
non-insulin-dependent diabetes. *See* type 2 diabetes

O'Keefe, Gail, 34, 64
oral medications, 50–51
    use of, vs. insulin, 62 (chart)
Orloff, David G., 14, 52
overweight/obesity
    in children, 13–14
    prevalence among type 2 diabetes, 45
    as risk factor for type 2 diabetes, 42
    surgery for, diabetes remission and, 77 (chart)
    type 2 diabetes epidemic and, 25

pancreas, 8, 9, 46 (illustration)
    artificial, 67
    drugs stimulating insulin production by, 50
    normal functioning of, 15–16
    numbers available for transplant, 76
    in type 1 vs. type 2 diabetes, 44
pancreatic-kidney transplants, 17, 66–67
    success of, 74
Peters, Anne L., 8, 28, 72
Phillipson, Louis, 70
Polonsky, William H., 23, 53
prediabetes
    growth in adults with, 31 (chart)
    prevention of diabetes in individuals with, 39
pregnancy, diabetes during. *See* gestational diabetes
prevention
    of diabetes, 7
    percent of health care spending devoted to, 74
    of type 1 diabetes, 18–19, 65–66
    of type 2 diabetes, 18, 64–65
prognosis, 6

Randy Jackson's Struggle with Diabetes (CBS News), 73
research, 7
    on beta cells, 69–70
    federal spending on, by disease area, 75 (table)
    importance of, 73
    on islet cells, 68–69
    on link between environment and genetics, 40
Ressler, Julie Ann, 56

Saudek, Christopher D., 66
Spiegel, Allen M., 65, 73
Spiro, Günther, 54
splenocytes, 68–69
Steinbrook, Robert, 28
sulfonylureas, 50
syndrome X. *See* metabolic syndrome

thiazolidinediones, 50
Thompson, Tommy, 21
Torres, Jaime, 18
type 1 diabetes, 35–36
    causes of, 44
    characteristics of, 47 (chart)
    groups at high risk for, 40
    prevention of, 18–19, 65–66
type 2 diabetes, 36–38
    in adults, as percent of all diabetes cases, 44
    characteristics of, 47 (chart)
    in children, 29
    diagnosis in children, 41
    epidemic of, 24–26
    groups at high risk for, 40
    importance of weight control in, 52
    obesity as risk factor for, 42
    prevention of, 18, 64–65

weight loss, 7
    insulin sensitivity and, 57
Wen, Li, 65
Westermark, Gunilla T., 68

Young, Andrew, 57

About the Author

Janice M. Yuwiler has a master's degree in public health and has spent over 15 years working to prevent children and adolescents from being injured. She is now working to ensure that children and adults needing social services or mental health get the help and support they need. Yuwiler has a background in epidemiology and molecular biology and delights in putting the latest science and medical breakthroughs in the hands of young people. Her other books include *Family Violence* and *Great Medical Discoveries: Insulin*. Yuwiler is a native Californian who enjoys living in sunny California with her husband and three children.

BAS 616.462 Yu929
Yuwiler, Janice.

Diabetes /
c2010.

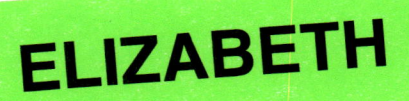

ELIZABETH